Adolescent Oral Health

Editor

DEBORAH STUDEN-PAVLOVICH

DENTAL CLINICS OF NORTH AMERICA

www.dental.theclinics.com

October 2021 • Volume 65 • Number 4

ELSEVIER

1600 John F. Kennedy Boulevard ● Suite 1800 ● Philadelphia, Pennsylvania, 19103-2899

http://www.dental.theclinics.com

DENTAL CLINICS OF NORTH AMERICA Volume 65, Number 4
October 2021 ISSN 0011-8532, ISBN: 978-0-323-84878-7

Editor: John Vassallo; j.vassallo@elsevier.com
Developmental Editor: Ann Gielou M. Posedio

Dental Clinics of North America (ISSN 0011-8532) is published quarterly by Elsevier Inc., 360 Park Avenue South, New York, NY 10010-1710. Months of issue are January, April, July, and October. Business and Editorial Offices: 1600 John F. Kennedy Boulevard, Suite 1800, Philadelphia, PA 19103-2899. Periodicals postage paid at New York, NY and additional mailing offices. Subscription prices are $313.00 per year (domestic individuals), $846.00 per year (domestic institutions), $100.00 per year (domestic students/residents), $366.00 per year (Canadian individuals), $888.00 per year (Canadian institutions), $100.00 per year (Canadian students/residents) $428.00 per year (international individuals), $888.00 per year (international institutions), and $200.00 per year (international students/residents). International air speed delivery is included in all *Clinics* subscription prices. All prices are subject to change without notice. **POSTMASTER:** Send address changes to *Dental Clinics of North America*, Elsevier Health Sciences Division, Subscription Customer Service, 3251 Riverport Lane, Maryland Heights, MO 63043. **Customer Service (orders, claims, online, change of address): Elsevier Health Sciences Division, Subscription Customer Service, 3251 Riverport Lane, Maryland Heights, MO 63043. Tel: 1-800-654-2452 (U.S. and Canada). Fax: 314-447-8029. E-mail: journalscustomerservice-usa@elsevier.com (for print support); journalsonlinesupport-usa@elsevier. com (for online support).**

Reprints. For copies of 100 or more, of articles in this publication, please contact the Commercial Reprints Department, Elsevier Inc., 360 Park Avenue South, New York, NY 10010-1710. Tel.: 212-633-3874; Fax: 212-633-3820; E-mail: reprints@elsevier.com.

The Dental Clinics of North America is covered in *MEDLINE/PubMed (Index Medicus), Current Contents/Clinical Medicine, ISI/BIOMED* and *Clinahl.*

Contributors

EDITOR

DEBORAH STUDEN-PAVLOVICH, DMD
Professor, Interim Chair, and Graduate Program Director, Department of Pediatric
Dentistry, University of Pittsburgh School of Dental Medicine, Pittsburgh, Pennsylvania

AUTHORS

DEANNA ADKINS, MD
Associate Professor, Division of Endocrinology and Metabolism, Department of
Pediatrics, Duke University School of Medicine, Durham, North Carolina

EDWARD C. ADLESIC, MS, DMD
Assistant Professor, Department of Oral and Maxillofacial Surgery, Assistant Professor,
Department of Dental Anesthesiology, University of Pittsburgh School of Dental Medicine,
Pittsburgh, Pennsylvania

MERT N. AKSU, DDS, JD, MHSA, Cert DPH
Dean and Professor, Diplomate, American Board of Dental Public Health, University of
Detroit Mercy, School of Dentistry, Detroit, Michigan

MATTHEW COOKE, DDS, MD, MPH
Associate Professor, Departments of Dental Anesthesiology, and Pediatric Dentistry,
University of Pittsburgh, School of Dental Medicine, Pittsburgh, Pennsylvania

MARCIO A. DA FONSECA, DDS, MS
Chicago Dental Society Foundation Professor and Head, Department of Pediatric
Dentistry, College of Dentistry, University of Illinois Chicago, Chicago, Illinois

MATTHEW DEMERLE, DDS, MD
Resident, Department of Oral and Maxillofacial Surgery, University of Pittsburgh Medical
Center, Pittsburgh, Pennsylvania

BRYCE HARTMAN, DDS
Former Chief Resident, Department of Oral and Maxillofacial Surgery, University of
Pittsburgh Medical Center, private practice, Pittsburgh, Pennsylvania

BRITTANEY HILL, DDS, MS, MPH
Clinical Assistant Professor, Department of Pediatric Dentistry, College of Dentistry,
University of Illinois Chicago, Chicago, Illinois

LEDA R.F. MUGAYAR, DDS, MS
Clinical Associate Professor, Department of Pediatric Dentistry, College of Dentistry,
University of Illinois Chicago, Chicago, Illinois

JOSHUA A. RAISIN, DDS
Resident and Graduate Teaching Assistant, Division of Pediatric and Public Health,
University of North Carolina Adams School of Dentistry, Chapel Hill, North Carolina

DENNIS N. RANALLI, DDS, MDS
Professor Emeritus, Department of Pediatric Dentistry, University of Pittsburgh, Senior Associate Dean Emeritus, School of Dental Medicine, University of Pittsburgh, Professor (Retired), Sports Medicine and Nutrition, School of Health and Rehabilitation Sciences, University of Pittsburgh, Pittsburgh, Pennsylvania

CAMERON L. RANDALL, PhD
Acting Assistant Professor, Department of Oral Health Sciences, University of Washington School of Dentistry, Seattle, Washington

HERBERT L. RAY Jr, DMD
Associate Professor, Chair and Graduate Program Director, Department of Endodontics, University of Pittsburgh School of Dental Medicine, Center for Craniofacial Regeneration, McGowan Institute for Regenerative Medicine, Pittsburgh, Pennsylvania

SCOTT B. SCHWARTZ, DDS, MPH
Assistant Professor, Department of Pediatrics, University of Cincinnati College of Medicine, Assistant Professor, Division of Pediatric Dentistry and Orthodontics, Cincinnati Children's Hospital Medical Center, Cincinnati, Ohio

MARK SOSOVICKA, DMD
Assistant Professor, Department of Oral and Maxillofacial Surgery, University of Pittsburgh School of Dental Medicine, Pittsburgh, Pennsylvania

DEBORAH STUDEN-PAVLOVICH, DMD
Professor, Interim Chair, and Graduate Program Director, Department of Pediatric Dentistry, University of Pittsburgh School of Dental Medicine, Pittsburgh, Pennsylvania

THOMAS TANBONLIONG, DDS
HS Associate Clinical Professor, Program Director, Postgraduate Pediatric Dentistry, Department of Orofacial Sciences, University of California San Francisco, School of Dentistry, San Francisco, California

JANICE A. TOWNSEND, DDS, MS
Chief, Department of Dentistry, Nationwide Children's Hospital, Chair and Associate Professor, Division of Pediatric Dentistry, The Ohio State University, Columbus, Ohio

ADRIANA MODESTO VIEIRA, DDS, MS, PhD, DMD
Professor, Assistant Dean of Diversity, Inclusion and Social Justice, Predoctoral Program Director, Department of Pediatric Dentistry, Department of Oral and Craniofacial Sciences, University of Pittsburgh School of Dental Medicine, Pittsburgh, Pennsylvania

KARIN WEBER-GASPARONI, DDS, MS, PhD
Professor and Chair, Department of Pediatric Dentistry, University of Iowa, Iowa City, Iowa

PAMELA ZARKOWSKI, JD, MPH
Provost and Vice President for Academic Affairs, Professor, School of Dentistry, University of Detroit Mercy, Office of Academic Administration, Detroit, Michigan

Contents

Preface: Current Perspectives in Adolescent Care   ix

Deborah Studen-Pavlovich

Oral Health Implications of Risky Behaviors in Adolescence   669

Brittaney Hill, Leda R.F. Mugayar, and Marcio A. da Fonseca

> Adolescence is a time for new discoveries, which may lead teens to engage in impulsive behaviors. Although social media and the Internet have brought great benefits to the world, they can also have a negative influence on adolescents, facilitating their engagement in risky behaviors. Positive parenting and healthy friendships in adolescence have a protective effect against sensation-seeking behaviors. Dental practitioners also have a significant role in steering young patients toward healthy behaviors. They play an essential role in the early recognition, initiation of appropriate interventions, and referrals for treatment of youth at risk.

Eating Disorders in the Adolescent Patient   689

Dennis N. Ranalli and Deborah Studen-Pavlovich

> Eating disorders such as anorexia nervosa, female athlete triad, bulimia nervosa, obesity, and binge eating initially emerge during adolescence. These disorders are present primarily in females, but males may also present with these conditions. Dentistry has a pivotal role in the management of patients with such diet-related disorders. Because dentists examine their patients at frequent intervals and may be the health care professionals with whom patients feel more comfortable discussing eating disorders, dentists must have knowledge of the etiology, diagnostic criteria, systemic effects, and intraoral manifestations of eating disorders. In addition, the dental professional may be the first health care provider to identify the condition and refer the patient appropriately to medical colleagues for subsequent treatment. This chapter provides dentists with current and relevant information to recognize, diagnose, and integrate dental treatment for their adolescent patients who may exhibit manifestations of an eating disorder.

Understanding and Caring for LGBTQ+ Youth by the Oral Health Care Provider   705

Joshua A. Raisin, Deanna Adkins, and Scott B. Schwartz

> With growing visibility, there is an increasing prevalence of lesbian, gay, bisexual, transgender, and queer (LGBTQ+) youth who feel empowered to own their true identity. Members of the oral health team frequently do not receive sufficient education in their training to recognize the nuance that treating this population may require. Although the tooth-level treatment does not materially change, a deeper appreciation of development of sexuality and gender identity, transgender medicine, and the health disparities LGBTQ+ youth face can promote more meaningful, trusting clinical relationships with this vulnerable population. This article aims to

provide members of the oral health team with the requisite knowledge to deliver culturally competent care to LGBTQ+ youth.

Transitioning Adolescent Patients with Special Health Care Needs from Pediatric to Adult Dental Care 719

Karin Weber-Gasparoni

Health care transition from adolescence into adulthood is a complex process that often lacks care coordination, planning, and collaboration among the parties involved. Dental transition is significantly more challenging for adolescents with special health care needs. Shortage of qualified general dentists willing to treat these individuals and low dental reimbursement by public insurance programs are significant barriers to successful transition. Adequate training to increase dental workforce, insurance benefits, protocol development, and research are needed to ensure successful transition for this population. Meanwhile, it is important to target individuals less likely to access adequate oral health care and achieve satisfactory transition.

Adolescent Dental Fear and Anxiety: Background, Assessment, and Nonpharmacologic Behavior Guidance 731

Janice A. Townsend and Cameron L. Randall

Adolescence, the period from 11 to 21 years of age, bridges the chasm between childhood and adulthood. Adolescence can be challenging as bodies, cognition, and personality go through major transformations, but it is also a time of great joy as confident adults with a clear identity develop. Dentists need to be knowledgeable about the developmental characteristics of this group because some of the cognitive and emotional changes make adolescents vulnerable to new fears. Dentists must tailor behavior guidance to this developing psyche in a way that respects independence and promotes confidence to foster lifelong positive views of dentistry.

Sedation and Anesthesia for the Adolescent Dental Patient 753

Matthew Cooke and Thomas Tanbonliong

This article focuses on sedation/anesthesia of adolescent patients in the dental setting. Preoperative evaluation, treatment planning, monitoring, and management are critical components to successful sedation. The authors discuss commonly administered agents and techniques to adolescents, including nitrous oxide/oxygen analgesia. The levels and spectrum of sedation and anesthesia are reviewed. Common comorbidities are also presented as they relate to sedation of the adolescent dental patient.

Pediatric Endodontic Treatment of Adolescent Patients 775

Adriana Modesto Vieira and Herbert L. Ray Jr.

This article is intended to familiarize clinicians with several pulp therapy modalities and new materials that are currently available for immature young pulp in the adolescent population. Objectives and considerations for immature young permanent teeth as well as the healing potential of the young pulp tissue after treatment of the inflammatory process are discussed. The article emphasizes that the future holds great possibilities for the regeneration of dental pulp in adolescent patients.

Adolescent Orofacial Trauma 787

Mark Sosovicka and Matthew DeMerle

Facial and dental-related trauma is common in the pediatric population. Appropriate evaluation and management techniques should be followed. Initial evaluation of the medical condition of the patient should be completed with acute management of any medical-related problems as a priority. ABCDEs of pediatric trauma should be followed and a thorough head and neck and oral examination completed with appropriate imaging if indicated. Newer dental trauma treatment protocols developed by the International Association of Dental Traumatology should be followed for best outcomes. Pediatric traumatic dental injuries generally have good prognosis by attempting to retain and stabilize teeth.

Evaluation and Management of Impacted Teeth in the Adolescent Patient 805

Bryce Hartman and Edward C. Adlesic

The most common oral and maxillofacial surgical procedure in adolescents is excision of impacted third molars. Adolescent patients should be evaluated for third molars starting around age 16 years unless symptomatic at an earlier age. The dental examination should include panorex imaging to assess development, pathologic condition, and possibility of eruption versus impaction. Various classification systems are available to identify the position and difficulty of the proposed surgical procedure. Retained impacted teeth increase the patient's risk of various morbidities including recurrent infection, damage to adjacent teeth, cysts and other lesions, and unexplained pain.

Legal and Ethical Issues in Treating Adolescent Patients 815

Pamela Zarkowski and Mert N. Aksu

Adolescent patients may present with unique and challenging ethical dilemmas and legal considerations during dental treatment. From the moment the patient registers with the practice, the issues of medical history, informed consent, treatment decisions, and role of the patient and parent affect the dynamic of the doctor-patient relationship. Providers are challenged with balancing the physical, psychological, and social changes occurring in these patients and the changing relationships between the patients and their parents/guardians. State laws, practice standards, and consumerism in dental practice all affect the relationship between the practice, the adolescent, and the parent/guardian.

DENTAL CLINICS OF NORTH AMERICA

FORTHCOMING ISSUES

January 2022
Biologics and Biology-based Regenerative Treatment Approaches in Periodontics
Alpdogan Kantarci, Andreas Stavropoulos, and Anton Sculean, *Editors*

April 2022
Special Care Dentistry
Stephanie M. Munz, *Editor*

July 2022
Smile Design
Behnam Bohluli, Shahrokh C Bagheri, and Omid Keyhan, *Editors*

RECENT ISSUES

July 2021
Radiographic Interpretation for the Dentist
Mel Mupparapu, *Editor*

April 2021
Geriatric Dental Medicine
Joseph M. Calabrese and Michelle Henshaw, *Editors*

January 2021
Implant Surgery
Harry Dym, *Editor*

SERIES OF RELATED INTEREST

Atlas of the Oral and Maxillofacial Surgery Clinics
http://www.oralmaxsurgeryatlas.theclinics.com

Oral and Maxillofacial Surgery Clinics
http://www.oralmaxsurgery.theclinics.com

THE CLINICS ARE AVAILABLE ONLINE!
Access your subscription at:
www.theclinics.com

Preface

Current Perspectives in Adolescent Care

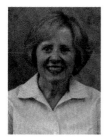

Deborah Studen-Pavlovich, DMD
Editor

In 2006, Dr Dennis N. Ranalli and I coedited the first issue of *Dental Clinics of North America* dedicated to adolescent oral health. At that time, journal articles and funded research were just beginning to emerge on the topics of adolescent health, and specifically, adolescent oral health. Following the first issue, we coauthored numerous articles on adolescent oral health, including body art, the adolescent athlete, and risky behaviors, among others. We had a strong interest in learning more about adolescent oral health and wished to convey that knowledge to other dentists and health care professionals. Since that first issue, there have been many trends and innovations affecting adolescent oral health, including the human papilloma virus vaccine, the increase in vaping by teenagers, and new techniques and products to treat orofacial trauma. These are some of the many reasons an updated issue on adolescent oral health was suggested by the publisher.

Adolescence is a stage of development in which many changes, physical, intellectual, and emotional, are all occurring simultaneously. It is a period in which the teenager is attempting to exert independence but may face difficulties along the way. The COVID-19 pandemic placed many difficulties on teens, social isolation, stress, and mental health issues. The dentist treating the adolescent patient needs to be aware of concerns and challenges confronting the adolescent. This updated issue addresses some of the areas currently affecting adolescent oral health.

The opening article discusses many of the risky behaviors often observed in teens that make them more vulnerable to trauma, disease, and other comorbidities. Eating disorders ranging from anorexia nervosa, the female athlete triad, bulimia, and to obesity all may affect adolescent oral health, as described in an article providing insight on how these conditions impact the orofacial complex. Development of a sexual identity, its conflicts, acceptance, and other issues, is described using current terminology, along with specific topics affecting LGBTQ+ adolescents.

Dent Clin N Am 65 (2021) ix–x
https://doi.org/10.1016/j.cden.2021.07.006
0011-8532/21/© 2021 Published by Elsevier Inc.

dental.theclinics.com

Patients with special health care needs often face difficulties during adolescence in securing a dentist who is adequately trained and capable of providing comprehensive dental care for them. The transition to adult care for these patients is an important topic addressed with meaningful recommendations.

Many adolescent patients lack the coping skills in adapting to the dental environment. One article in this current issue evaluates nonpharmacologic approaches to address this concern and offers psychological methods for adaptation. If nonpharmacologic methods are ineffective, sedation modalities are explored in a subsequent article. Recommendations for safe and effective pharmacosedation are offered for the dentist.

Dental trauma and caries are more frequent during adolescence with both of these insults to the dentition being seen by dentists routinely. Current endodontic knowledge of the treatments available and the preferred medicaments are presented concisely in an article.

Since orofacial trauma affects adolescents far more often than younger children, in-depth knowledge of stabilization of the patient, evaluating facial fractures, soft tissue management, and dentoalveolar injuries are presented in another article. Impacted permanent third molars may pose a concern during late adolescence. The authors covering this topic present pertinent information on evaluation, the pros and cons of preserving the teeth or extracting them, and other guidance useful for the practitioner.

Although many adolescents may appear to be adults based on their physical appearance, they may not be permitted to consent for dental treatment depending on the state where they reside. Being aware of emancipation definitions, emergent situations, guardianship, and informed consent is an important issue for the practitioner, as addressed in an article regarding legal issues.

The dentist must have the requisite knowledge of adolescent oral health concerns and be able to apply the concepts of anticipatory guidance to the adolescent's dental care. My coauthors and I hope that you will find the information within this issue helpful and incorporate the knowledge and practical guidance into your practices.

Deborah Studen-Pavlovich, DMD
Department of Pediatric Dentistry
University of Pittsburgh School of Dental Medicine
366A Salk Hall
3501 Terrace Street
Pittsburgh, PA 15261, USA

E-mail address:
das12@pitt.edu

Oral Health Implications of Risky Behaviors in Adolescence

Brittaney Hill, DDS, MS, MPH, Leda R.F. Mugayar, DDS, MS,
Marcio A. da Fonseca, DDS, MS*

KEYWORDS

• Adolescent • Oral health • Health risk behavior • Internet • Illicit substances

KEY POINTS

- Alcohol was the most frequently used substance by high school students in the United States in 2019.
- Ninety percent of adults who smoke cigarettes daily tried it first before the age of 18 years.
- Electronic cigarettes ("vaping") is now the most common tobacco product used by youth.
- Most adolescents in the United States engage in some form of substance use during high school.
- After legalization in many American states, adolescent use of cannabis has increased, under the perception that it is socially acceptable and safer than alcohol and other drugs.

INTRODUCTION

Adolescence is a time for new discoveries and independence, and the uneven maturation of the young brain may lead adolescents to engage in impulsive and risky behaviors. Social media and the Internet have brought great benefits to the world, but they can also be a negative influence on adolescents, facilitating their engagement in such behaviors, many times protected by the anonymity and secrecy the Internet allows. Despite facilitating a faster connection with the world, heavy use of the Internet may also promote social isolation, depression, and suicidal ideation. It has also led to the appearance of a new disorder called Internet Gaming Disorder (IGD), which will be discussed in this article. Positive parenting and healthy friendships in early adolescence are crucial to reducing risky behaviors. Thus, household rules regarding early exposure to drinking, smoking, and recreational drugs, as well as excessive Internet use and video game playing, have a protective effect on youth that may last a lifetime.

Department of Pediatric Dentistry, College of Dentistry, University of Illinois Chicago, 801 South Paulina Street, Suite 250 (MC-850), Chicago, IL 60612, USA
* Corresponding author.
E-mail address: marcio@uic.edu

Dental providers can also play an important mentorship role for adolescents. They have a significant role in the early recognition, initiation of appropriate interventions, and referrals for the treatment of youth at risk. Although most dental professionals may not feel prepared to talk about sensitive topics with their patients, they are essential to understand the patients' and families' ability to follow-up with oral care recommendations. On the contrary, most patients are not aware of the oral-systemic health connections and may refrain from disclosing important health and psychosocial information that could lead to better oral health outcomes. Understanding social determinants of health is a tenet of contemporary dental practice that cannot be ignored. Dental practitioners must also familiarize themselves with local laws about adolescent rights to privacy and confidentiality before disclosing sensitive information that may not be shared with parents.

This article will discuss several risky behaviors of adolescents and their implications for oral health. Data shown are for youth in the United States (US), unless otherwise noted.

DISCUSSION
Tobacco and Electronic Cigarettes

Tobacco use remains the leading cause of preventable disease and death in the US.[1,2] Tobacco use is most commonly adopted during adolescence, when the brain is most vulnerable to nicotine addiction and when life-long habits are likely to be formed.[1,2] Therefore, it is important to recognize and address the detrimental impact that tobacco use can have on an adolescent's oral and general health.[1,2] Research has shown that 90% of adults who smoke cigarettes daily tried their first cigarette before the age of 18 years.[2] Although the current use (ie, within the past 30 days) of any tobacco product among middle and high school students decreased from 2017 to 2019, there were still almost 4.5 million youth tobacco users in 2020.[3] Ubiquitous advertising and influence of social media make adolescents more likely to try new and traditional tobacco products.

Tobacco products used by adolescents include cigarettes, electronic cigarettes (e-cigarettes), cigars, smokeless tobacco, heated tobacco products, hookah, and pipe tobacco. The current use of cigarettes among middle and high school students has decreased over the past 9 years. In 2020, 6.2% of them reported current cigarette use, down from 15.1% in 2011.[3–6] It is predicted that if cigarette smoking among young people continues at the current rate, 5.6 million US youth will die early from a smoking-related illness.[1] Since 2014, e-cigarettes ("vaping") have been the most common tobacco product used by adolescents in the US, especially with the availability of multiple flavors. In 2020, 24.3% of middle and high school students reported current e-cigarette use,[3] but it was down from 38% in 2019, when vaping among adolescents increased dramatically.[4,5] After e-cigarettes, the next most commonly used tobacco product by young students is cigars. In 2020, 6.5% of them reported current cigar use, which was 8.6% less than what they reported in 2011.[3–6] Smokeless tobacco use by youth has also decreased over the past 9 years. In 2020, only 4.2% of middle and high school students reported current use, down from 10.1% in 2011.[3–6] Almost 3% of those students reported current use of heated tobacco.[3] Hookah was the only product that showed no decrease in current use among students from 2011 to 2020 (5%).[3–6] Pipe tobacco was the least used tobacco product by youth in 2020 (1.1%).[3]

Many young people use more than two tobacco products, making them more likely to develop nicotine addiction and more likely to continue use well into adulthood.[1,7] In 2020, 11% of middle and high school students reported current use of two or more tobacco products.[3,5] Numerous factors influence the use of tobacco products during adolescence, including the physical and social environment in which they reside. Youth living with parents who use tobacco, those with friends who use tobacco products, and high school athletes are more likely to use these products than their peers.[2,7,8] Youth are also more likely to use tobacco products if they are from lower socioeconomic status households, have caregivers who are less attentive or supportive, have low self-esteem, and if they suffer from mental health issues, such as anxiety, depression, and stress.[2,7,8] Therefore, it is extremely important to develop targeted interventions that will reduce and prevent the use of tobacco products among adolescents.

Oral health implications
The use of tobacco can have both short and long-term adverse effects on oral and systemic health. Cigarette smoking has been linked to about 90% of all lung cancer cases, the leading cause of cancer-related death in both men and women.[9] Tobacco use is also associated with oral cancer, cancer of the pharynx, larynx, esophagus, stomach, pancreas, cervix, kidney, and bladder.[9] The use of tobacco drastically increases the risk for pulmonary and cardiovascular diseases, such as coronary heart disease, which is the leading cause of death in the US.[9]

All forms of tobacco currently available on the market have oral health consequences. Smoking cigarettes can lead to gingival recession, impaired healing after periodontal therapy, periodontal disease, mucosal lesions, tooth staining, and oral cancer.[10,11] Smokeless tobacco can cause gingival keratosis, gingival recession, periodontal disease, tooth loss, halitosis, alveolar bone damage, and dental caries because of sugars that may be added to the products.[10,11] Nicotine, the primary addicting component of tobacco products, can also lead to local burning sensation, throat irritation, dry lips, and ulcerations.[12]

Illicit Drug Use

National US surveys show that most adolescents engage in some form of substance use during high school.[13] Illicit substance use in adolescence is strongly associated with misuse by friends outside school, boyfriend/girlfriend, siblings, and online friends, which shows the impact of peer influence.[14] Besides that, other risk factors for illicit drug use include social disadvantages, limited parental monitoring, parental substance use, impulsive personality, poor school performance, easy access to alcohol and other substances, and affiliation with delinquent peers.[13,15] The progression from alcohol and tobacco to cannabis and later to other illicit substances is clear.[15,16] In the US, legalization of medical marijuana in certain states has led to more use of crack/cocaine and heroin by youth.[17]

The past decade saw a decrease in alcohol consumption by US youth but increased use of e-cigarettes, marijuana, and opioids.[18] The 2009 to 2019 survey of substance use behaviors of US high school students also showed a decrease in the prevalence of lifetime use of marijuana, cocaine, methamphetamine, heroin, synthetic marijuana, and injection drug use.[13] Of particular concern are the lifetime rate (1 in 7 adolescents) and current prevalence (1 in 14) of opioid misuse; those students also showed high rates of misuse of other substances.[13] In 2019, 29.2% of students used alcohol, 21.7% consumed marijuana, 13.7% reported binge drinking, and 7.2% misused prescription opioids.[13] Boys had a higher prevalence of lifetime use of cocaine, methamphetamine, heroin, and injection drug use while girls abused alcohol and prescription opioids more often.[13] Black and Hispanic students misused prescription opioids more frequently than whites, who had a higher prevalence of alcohol consumption.[13] Lesbian, gay, and bisexual students had a higher prevalence of all substance use behaviors, except binge drinking, compared with heterosexual students.[13]

Cannabis is a broad term used to describe the different products, such as marijuana and cannabinoids, that are derived from the cannabis sativa plant.[19] Its use has increased in recent years, possibly due to the legalization in certain states and the rise in its social acceptance.[20] Historically, cannabis had been smoked as marijuana; however, it has become increasingly available in a variety of forms, including edibles and topically applied products.[19] Although recreational marijuana use by adolescents is not legal in any US state, they continue to use it, under the perception that it is safer than alcohol and other drugs.[21] There are no significant differences in marijuana used based on gender, race/ethnicity, grade in school, or sexual identity.[13,21]

Frequent cannabis use has been associated with chronic systemic health effects, including addiction, difficulty thinking and problem solving, problems with memory, and impaired coordination.[22,23] It may also be associated with psychotic disorders and an increase in psychotic symptoms.[24] Cannabis contains many of the same carcinogens as tobacco, therefore repeated use can also lead to cardiovascular and respiratory pathologies.[25] With the documented detrimental effects that cannabis can have on the adolescent brain and other body systems, it is imperative that dental professionals participate in the provision of anticipatory guidance to help decrease its use among this population.

Abuse of cannabis rarely leads to death, in contrast to opioids and other illicit drugs.[15] These substances can also cause mental health issues, chronic health problems, and high-risk behaviors that can lead to pregnancy, sexually transmitted diseases (STDs, such as human immunodeficiency virus [HIV], human papillomavirus [HPV], etc.), exposure to coronavirus, motor vehicle accidents (MVAs), suicidal ideation, homicides, and violence.[13,15]

Oral health implications

The use of cannabis, particularly marijuana smoking, is associated with poor oral health; however, determining the etiology of the oral health problems can be complicated because of additional risky behaviors of those who are frequent users. Adolescents who engage in marijuana use may also use tobacco, alcohol, and other illegal substances, which have their own oral health consequences. Cannabis use has been linked to xerostomia, thus it contributes to an increased caries incidence.[26–28] Cannabis can also be an appetite stimulant, leading to higher consumption of foods and snacks that may be cariogenic.[29,30] This can be particularly detrimental during adolescence, when patients are also more likely to be inattentive to oral hygiene practices, have heightened caries experience, and gaps in oral health care access.

Smoking marijuana is also associated with gingival enlargement, erythroplakia, chronic inflammation of the oral mucosa with hyperkeratosis, and leukoplakia, which has the potential to become malignant.[26–28] Cancer associated with cannabis use is more aggressive in younger users, and those who use both tobacco and cannabis are at an increased risk for oral and neck cancer.[26,31,32] Cannabis use has been linked to periodontal disease, with higher rates of periodontitis being observed among frequent users than nonusers.[33,34] Chronic periodontitis may occur at an earlier age in marijuana users, which is especially important to note when counseling adolescents about marijuana use.[34–36]

Patients on cannabis may also present behavioral challenges for the dental provider. Cannabis use can cause anxiety, paranoia, hallucinations, and hyperactivity, which can make patients more stressed during their dental appointments.[26,27,37] It can also cause increased heart rate and other cardiac effects that could make the administration of local anesthesia with epinephrine and other anxiolytic agents potentially dangerous.[27,37,38] Patients, especially those who are under the legal buying age, may be unwilling to self-report cannabis use; therefore, it is important that dental providers are aware of the signs and symptoms of cannabis use. Owing to the risk of medical emergencies when treating intoxicated patients, practitioners should postpone nonemergent treatment in those situations.

To prevent misuse of prescription drugs by youth, dentists must reduce the number of prescriptions and the amount in the prescription as well as participate in prescription drug monitoring programs.[13,18] They must also consider the drug-seeking behavior of addicted legal guardians who may use the adolescent to obtain prescription drugs for their own use. Illicit substances can also interact with general anesthetics; thus, careful preoperative evaluation is crucial for safe delivery of care and alleviating the effects of drug withdrawal.[39,40] Other harmful effects of illicit drugs in the oral cavity include bruxism, tooth wear, lip paresthesia, ulcers, trismus, and temporomandibular joint dislocation.[41–45] To alleviate xerostomia, many individuals use soft drinks or sports drinks to quench their thirst, increasing their caries and dental erosion risk.[41] These patients should receive supplemental fluoride in the form of mouth rinses, toothpastes with high concentration of fluoride and more frequent professional applications.

Driving and Sports Safety

Adolescent driving

MVAs are the second leading cause of death for teens in the US.[46] In 2018, 2500 teens aged 13 to 19 years were killed and 285,000 were treated in emergency departments for injuries suffered as a result of MVAs.[46] Individuals aged between 16 and 19 years were almost 3 times more likely to be involved in a fatal crash than those aged more than 20 years.[47] Men, teens driving with other teen passengers in the car, and newly licensed teens are at especially high risk for motor vehicle crashes.[48–50] In 2019, 2,375 teenagers aged 13-19 years died in a car crash; 2 out of 3 were males.[47]

Seat belt use is essential to prevent casualties from MVAs; however, teens and young adults have the lowest seat belt use rates.[51] In 2019, 43% of high school students in the US reported they did not always wear a seatbelt when riding with someone else.[52] In 2019, half of teenage drivers who died in a car crash were not wearing a seat belt.[47] Driving while distracted, such as sending a text message, talking on the telephone, using a navigation system, and/or eating, also puts young drivers at higher risk for MVAs.[52] In 2019, 39% of high school students who drove in the past 30 days texted or emailed while driving on at least 1 day.[52] Those who texted and emailed while driving were also more likely to report they did not wear a seatbelt, were more likely to ride with a driver who had been drinking alcohol, and more likely to drive after drinking alcohol.[53]

Drinking any amount of alcohol before driving also increases accident risk among teen drivers.[47,54] In 2019, 5.4% of driving high school students reported that they had been drinking alcohol at least once before driving within the previous 30 days.[52] Drinking and driving were higher for students who were older, men, Hispanic, and with lower grades.[52] Students who engaged in other transportation risk behaviors (ie, speeding, distracted driving, etc.) were up to 30 times more likely to drive after consuming alcohol.[52] Teen drivers have a much higher risk for being involved in a crash than adult drivers with the same blood alcohol concentration (BAC).[54] They are also more likely to be involved in accidents when they have BAC levels below the legal limit for adults.[54]

Speeding also puts adolescent drivers at higher risk for MVAs. In 2018, 30% of male drivers and 18% of female drivers aged between 15 and 20 years who were involved in fatal crashes were speeding.[53] Teen drivers are more likely to speed in general and less likely to keep the appropriate distance between cars while driving compared with older drivers.[53]

The adolescent athlete

It is important that caregivers and adolescent athletes recognize the risk of participating in sports as well as the importance of taking the appropriate safety measures to prevent injury. Besides preventing trauma to the oral cavity during athletic activities, caregivers and medical/dental providers must also be aware of other risky behaviors in which the adolescent athlete might engage. For example, they may strive to achieve optimal weight and physical qualities to make them competitive, which could cause disordered eating and eventually an eating disorder. The prevalence of disordered eating and eating disorders in adolescent athletes is high, especially those competing in weight-sensitive sports.[55] This frequently occurs because of the desire to achieve the "ideal" body and to alleviate body dissatisfaction.[55]

Adolescent athletes are also likely to drink alcohol, use tobacco, steroids, and other performance-enhancing substances.[56–58] Highly active athletes are more likely to drink excessively than their peers, especially male athletes.[56–58] Early use of steroids and other performance-enhancing substances are also an area of concern. This is most commonly seen in men and non-Hispanic whites, and tends to occur earlier in athletes than their peers.[57] Steroid use also varies based on the type of sport, being more common among those involved in strength training sports like gymnastics and football.[57] Youth participation in sports has been associated with higher odds of binge drinking and e-cigarette smoking, but with lower odds of cannabis and cigarette use.[58,59] Young cigarette smokers tend to be more sedentary than e-cigarette users.[59]

Athletes, their families, and athletic personnel must also be aware of the proper safety measures and management protocols related to concussions. Sport-related concussions can interfere with schoolwork, social interactions, and prevent participation in sports.[60] If undiagnosed and/or untreated, long-term cognitive impairments may occur.[60]

Oral health implications

Orofacial trauma can be an outcome of MVAs and sport-related accidents. In addition to medical assessments and treatment, individuals involved in any type of accident should be evaluated for possible dental, oral, and facial bones–related injuries. Medical and dental providers must be aware of the protocol for the management of dental trauma and should treat emergent cases and/or make referrals to other specialists, especially in cases involving craniofacial structures other than the teeth.

Although physical injury during MVAs and sports accidents may be inevitable, taking the necessary precautions, such as wearing seatbelts and protective sports equipment (mouth guards, helmets, etc.) is of great importance. Traumatic dental injuries resulting from participation in sports as well as in leisure activities, such as skateboarding, roller-skating, and bicycling, have been significantly decreased by wearing well-fitting mouth guards and protective equipment.[61–64] When accidents do occur, timely management of orofacial trauma is very important, as the long-term effects can lead to prolonged treatment needs, difficulties with speech, eating, and a negative impact on oral health-related quality of life.[64]

Disordered eating, eating disorders, and use of tobacco cause negative impacts on oral health, which have been discussed in this and other articles in this issue. Athletes may also attempt to maintain proper hydration by consuming isotonic beverages, which can increase caries risk because of high sugar content and cause enamel erosion because of their acidic pH.[65] There is also a connection between enamel erosion and prolonged exposure to chlorinated swimming pool water in competitive swimmers.[66] Therefore, dental professionals must give clear recommendations to athletes to prevent dental trauma, caries, and erosion.

Alcohol Use

Alcohol was the most frequently used substance by US high school students in 2019 (29.2%).[13] The prevalence of current alcohol use was higher for women, and for white (34.2%) and Hispanic students (28.4%) more than black students (16.8%).[13] Several factors may lead an adolescent to early alcohol use. Regular smoking and social anxiety disorder are known predictive factors for early use of alcohol.[67] Parental alcohol use disorder (AUD) is also a consistent predictor of increased early use of alcohol, cannabis, and sexual initiation of their offspring.[68] In addition to that, adolescents' exposure to alcohol on media and other means (eg, movies) is correlated with their initiation of drinking alcohol as well as increased drinking among those already using it.[69] Most importantly, early initiation of alcohol use, including binge drinking and heavy drinking, predicts AUD later in life.[67,70,71]

Binge drinking is defined as alcohol consumption that raises the BAC to at least 0.08% (ie, 5 drinks for men and 4 for women within 2 hours), whereas heavy drinking uses the same criterion but in a higher frequency (5 or more days in the last 30 days).[70] Binge drinking is the most common pattern of alcohol consumption in adolescents and young adults,[70] being reported by 13.7% of US high school students in 2019, with women showing substantially higher rates than men (31.9% vs 26.4%).[13] Both binge and heavy drinking cause neurobiological changes, affecting brain responses in several regions while performing a variety of tasks, including risky decision-making (eg, having unprotected sex, driving after drinking, using illicit substances, etc.) and reward response.[70] It may also lead them to more exposure to the current coronavirus.

Changes in alcohol consumption among college students because of the COVID-19 pandemic have been documented. College students who moved from living with peers to parents showed greater decrease in drinking days, number of drinks per week, and maximum drinks in 1 day than those who remained living with friends or were already living with parents.[72] Thus, returning to live with parents during early adulthood may be protective against heavy drinking.[72]

Oral health implications

The increased risk for oral diseases in individuals who abuse alcohol depends on their age and the length of alcohol addiction. A Ukrainian study found that the prevalence rate of oral diseases for 14- to 17-year-old individuals who had been abusing alcohol for 2 years was 10.9%, and 16.8% for those who had abused it for 3 years.[73] Thus, assessment of the oral status in young alcohol abusers is of great clinical significance for early detection of diseases of the oral mucosa, including potential precancerous lesions.

The cytotoxic effect of alcohol is among the leading causes of malignant degeneration of the oral mucosa.[73] The toxic effect of ethanol and/or its metabolite acetaldehyde on the oral mucosa results in increased cell regeneration that may play an important role in tumor promotion.[74] Chronic ethanol consumption causes oral mucosa atrophy, which may result in an enhanced susceptibility of the mucosal epithelium to chemical carcinogens, thus creating a major risk factor for oral and pharyngeal cancer.[73] Alcohol breaks down into acetaldehyde, which can bind to the proteins in the oral cavity triggering an inflammatory response in the body, causing the development of cancerous cells.[74]

Alcohol consumption is associated with increased occurrence of periodontitis due to impairment of neutrophil function, leading to bacterial overgrowth that may cause periodontal inflammation.[74,75] In addition to that, alcohol may have a toxic effect on periodontal tissue and may increase monocyte production of inflammatory cytokines in the gingival crevice, which is associated with periodontitis and attachment loss.[74]

Features suggestive of alcohol misuse include missed dental appointments, alcoholic breath, parotid gland enlargement, glossitis, loss of tongue papillae, spider angiomas, and angular cheilitis caused by malnutrition.[76,77] Teens who abuse alcohol also tend to present with more dental trauma.[78,79] The dental professional should stress the importance of daily oral hygiene and a healthy diet as they are not usually a priority for these patients. Invasive dental procedures should only be done when the individual is stable.[76] Consultation with the patient's physician is a necessity to discuss drug selection and administration as well as potential bleeding tendencies.[76]

The use of a single alcohol screening question is ideal for the dental practitioner because it is simple and not time-consuming. Providers should ask male patients if they have consumed 5 or more standard drinks on one occasion in the past year (4 drinks for a woman). A positive answer may indicate an alcohol problem, requiring a more detailed evaluation by the primary care physician.[76]

Internet Addiction, Internet Gaming Disorder, and Gambling

Internet addiction, IGD, and gambling are growing concerns related to risky behaviors in adolescence. Internet addiction and problematic *Facebook* use are significant global problems that can lead to somatic and mental symptoms, such as depression, psychoticism, paranoid ideation, suicidal ideation and attempts, anxiety, and serious mental illness.[80–82] It has also been linked to withdrawal from sports and clubs, alcohol abuse, attention deficit, and hyperactivity.[81,83] However, some authors consider excessive use of the Internet as a symptom of mental health problems rather than a cause.[81]

The fifth version of the *Diagnostic and Statistical Manual of Mental Disorders* added IGD, which also includes non-Internet gaming sources, as a potential new diagnosis because heavy gaming can cause psychosocial and medical problems.[84] Risk factors for IGD include male sex, young age, and psychological symptoms, such as depression and social isolation.[84] Gaming is particularly attractive to those in social isolation or with poor interpersonal skills because it allows them to develop online relationships and assume new personalities.[84] Impulsivity has also been linked to IGD and can lead to risky behaviors, such as smoking, drug use, and violence.[84,85] Excessive gaming may also alter the brain in a way that it increases the risk of depression and aggressive behavior.[85] In addition to that, pathologic video game use can lead to poor school grades and attention problems.[86] Students who are heavy Internet users, whether they are gamers or not, show similar higher risks for emotional problems, conduct disorder, hyperactivity, inattention, self-injurious behaviors, and suicidal ideation.[86]

Social media also seems to be a major global influencer on youth gambling. A strong sense of belonging to an online community is associated with higher problem gambling, especially if adolescents are involved in social media identity bubbles.[87] Regular gambling by adolescents and young adults has been associated with parental gambling behavior, maternal educational background, cigarette smoking, misuse of alcohol, illicit drug use, suicide attempts, and fighting.[87–91] Other risk factors include male sex, low educational attainment, low socioeconomic status, unemployment, sensation seeking, cyberbullying, and delinquency.[91–93] Problematic gambling also includes lottery games, scratch cards, card games, and sports betting.[91]

Oral health implications

There are no studies to date linking specific oral health issues to Internet addiction, gaming, and gambling. However, as these adolescents may develop psychological issues that can lead to risky behaviors and sensation seeking, there is a potential for behavioral problems in the dental office as well as oral manifestations of substance use and STDs. Furthermore, these adolescents may not prioritize diet and oral hygiene, which may lead to increased risk for obesity, caries, and periodontal disease.

Human (Adolescent) Trafficking

Human trafficking includes sex trafficking, labor trafficking (domestic work, agriculture, farming, etc.), or sex and labor trafficking combined (prostitution, working in bars and strip clubs, etc.).[94] Adolescent sex trafficking is defined as the recruitment, harboring, transportation, provision, obtaining, patronizing, or soliciting of a minor for the purpose of a commercial sexual act.[95] No youth is safe from becoming a trafficking victim, regardless of race, age, socioeconomic status, or location (urban, suburban or rural, or country of origin).[95,96] International victims usually come from countries torn by poverty, or political and economic instability.[95]

The United States has a homegrown problem of youth being exploited for commercial sex.[95] Adolescents who come from poor or minority families, runaways, those involved with the child welfare system or juvenile justice, victims of physical abuse, sexual abuse or abandonment, undocumented immigrants, and those addicted to drugs and/or alcohol are the typical targets of pimps and traffickers.[94,95,97] Other risk factors include having family members in sex work and having friends who sold or bought sex.[97] Pimps and traffickers attract victims with offers of food, shelter, employment, love, friendship, nice clothes, jewelry, and a better life prospect, moving them away from families and friends.[94,95] They use emotional, physical, and psychological abuse to keep victims trapped in a life of prostitution or forced labor.[95] Eventually, these adolescents will suffer from depression, feelings of hopelessness, and low self-esteem.[95]

Health care providers, including dental professionals, frequently overlook or fail to identify trafficked youth, resulting in continued perpetration of crimes against them.[96] One of the reasons is their lack of education and comfort in discussing the topic. Stereotypes may also prevent them from recognizing as victims patients who are already under their care, such as US citizens, those from high socioeconomic classes and boys.[96] However, recognizing trafficking victims can be challenging. Some red flags include individuals who lack proper documentation; who lie about their age; who are accompanied by someone who is older, not a relative or legal guardian (eg, boyfriend), and/or who is very controlling and does not leave the person alone; those who give inconsistent histories to explain their health condition or chief complaint; individuals who do not have a medical or dental home; who wear expensive clothing and jewelry that do not seem appropriate; and who carry large amounts of cash.[98,99] Many victims do not self-disclose even if they have the opportunity, fearing for their safety and that of family members, or because they feel ashamed or hopeless about their situation.[95,96,98,100] Observing the patient's body language and other visual cues, as well as their communication style and that of the accompanying person, can aid in the identification or suspicion of victims.[99]

Oral health implications

One important aspect of providing health care to individuals involved in traumatic situations, such as sexual abuse and trafficking, is through trauma-informed care (TIC). TIC is defined as "understanding, respecting, and appropriately responding to how human trafficking and other types of trauma affect a survivor's life, behavior, and sense of themselves."[101] That means providing a safe environment for the patient (trained staff on the issue, confidentiality, reporting procedures, etc.), using an interpreter other than the person accompanying the patient, trying to provide a private environment for interviews and treatment (separate the patient from the accompanying person), and being aware of how medical and dental care can retraumatize a victim, among others.[101] The dentist, or any auxiliary staff, may be able to separate the patient from the accompanying person by taking the patient away for a radiograph or simply stating that office policy dictates that the examination be done privately.[100] If the dentist believes the patient is a trafficking victim, the *National Human Trafficking Resource Center* hotline (1-888-373-7888) can be contacted for help.[94] If the victim refuses assistance, the provider should give him/her the hotline number and in case of minors, a report must be filed with the child protection services.

The trafficking victim may have dental and oral problems because of neglect and/or dental trauma. The oral health professional must take a detailed health history, particularly concerning STDs, mental health issues (post-traumatic stress disorder, anxiety, substance abuse, panic disorder, depression, etc.), tuberculosis, malnutrition, pregnancy, and physical injuries.[95,96] Trafficking victims may also be more exposed to the novel coronavirus and have less access to testing and treatment.

Sexual Behavior

Preventing unintended pregnancy and STDs among adolescents is a public health priority. In 2015% to 2017%, 42% of female teenagers and 38% of male adolescents in the US were sexually active,[102] with non-Hispanic black male teens showing higher rates of sexual activity than Hispanics and non-white Hispanics.[103] Condoms are the most commonly used contraceptive method among US teens (97%).[102] Other frequently used methods include withdrawal (65%), oral contraceptives (53%), long-acting reversible contraception (20%), and emergency contraception (19%).[102] Non-white Hispanics presented higher percentages of using any contraceptive method than Hispanics and blacks.[103] In the US, there is greater reliance on condom use and withdrawal than other contraceptive methods because adolescents either do not have health insurance or are covered by their parents' insurance plan, leading to confidentiality issues.[104]

There is a growing concern about the increase in the prevalence of STDs in adolescents, specifically between 15 and 19 years of age.[105] Several factors account for the increase—teens are more likely to engage in high-risk sexual behavior, less likely to use sexual health services, whereas female teens have lower production of cervical mucous and increased cervical ectopy, which facilitates the development of STDs.[105] One in four sexually active female teenagers aged between 15 and 19 years in the US has an STD, especially chlamydia and HPV.[105] These diseases can cause chronic health problems if not treated early or if left untreated. They can lead to nervous system and cardiovascular system damage (due to tertiary syphilis), adverse birth outcomes and infertility (gonorrhea), cervical, oropharyngeal and rectal cancers (HPV), and acquired immunodeficiency syndrome (HIV).[105] The HPV vaccine introduced in 2006 has led to a 64% reduction in HPV prevalence among women from 14 to 19 years of age and became a critical component of teenage sexual health due to high vaccine effectiveness.[105] HPV vaccine is recommended for 11 and 12-year-old boys and girls, with catch-up vaccination up to 26 years of age.[106]

Adolescents are more likely to engage in oral sex than intercourse, report more oral sex partners than intercourse partners, and unlikely to use STD protection during oral sex,[106,107] which has led to a significant increase in the prevalence of genital HSV-1.[105,106] Other populations at high risk for STDs include homeless, incarcerated or drug-using youth.[105]

Another significant concern is an unplanned pregnancy. In the US, the number of births to teen mothers has dropped steadily since 1990, declining 45% from 2001 to 2013.[104] In 2018, just under 180,000 infants were born to 15- to 19-year-old teens.[108] This lower trend has been driven both by fewer teenagers having sex and more birth control use.[104,108,109]

Oral health implications

Screening and examination for oral signs of STDs and appropriate referral by the dental provider are important because STDs frequently affect the mucous membranes producing characteristic lesions on the oral mucosa. HPV can affect the mouth and throat, and some high-risk strains, particularly HPV-16, are associated with cancers of the head and neck.[105,106,110] These cancers are four times more common in men than in women and tend to develop at the base of the tongue, in the folds of the tonsils or the back of the throat, making them difficult to detect.[110,111] Low risk strains of HPV may cause warts or lesions in the mouth or throat.[105,111] Aside from their appearance, they often have very few symptoms, which are painless and noncancerous. They can reappear from time to time, and they should be surgically removed.[110] Therefore, dental professionals are in a unique position to discuss HPV prevention and vaccination with their patients and parents.

There are two strains of HSV and there is no cure for either one.[111] HSV-1 is most commonly associated with cold sores and other oral lesions, whereas HSV-2 is associated with genital lesions.[111] Both strains are extremely contagious and can be passed between the genitals and the mouth through saliva and contact with open sores during and right before an outbreak.[111] During an outbreak, blisters will appear in the mouth, which generally heal within 7 to 10 days.[111] Analgesics can be prescribed to reduce fever and pain and antiviral drugs, such as acyclovir and valacyclovir, can be effective for the treatment of herpes as well as cold sores.[111]

Syphilis may appear as sores (chancres) on the lips, tip of the tongue, gingiva, or at the back of the mouth near the tonsils in the first stages of infection.[112] They start as small red patches and grow into large open sores that can be red, yellow, or gray in color, which are very contagious and often painful.[112] Although oral manifestations can be observed at the primary stage, they are more commonly detected at the secondary stage as multiple painless ulcers with irregularly shaped whitish edges on the oral mucosa, tongue, lips, and buccal mucosa.[112] The sores may resolve even if untreated, but the individual still may have syphilis and can infect others.[112] The dental provider can do a biopsy to confirm the diagnosis. If positive, a referral to the patient's primary care physician for more testing and treatment should be done.

Gonorrhea is a bacterial infection that affects mucous membranes, including those in the mouth and throat.[110] It can be difficult to detect because its symptoms are often very mild and can go unnoticed. The most common oral symptoms are soreness or burning in the throat, but swollen glands and occasionally white spots in the mouth might also occur.[110] Pharyngitis is often asymptomatic but may manifest with an exudative sore throat.[110] A throat culture swab test can diagnose gonorrhea if symptoms in the mouth are present.

SUMMARY

Most adolescents engage in some form of substance use during high school and may potentially develop addictions from that experience. No youth is safe; even athletes, who tend to be very healthy, can fall victim to smoking, drinking, use of illicit substances, and early use of steroids. The legalization of cannabis in certain states has led to the rise in its social acceptance and the perception that it is safe, which has attracted more teens to use it. Furthermore, the progression from alcohol and tobacco to cannabis and later to other illicit substances is clearly demonstrated in many studies. The US also has a homegrown problem of youth being exploited for commercial sex, and no teen is safe from becoming a victim.

Youth living with parents who use tobacco, alcohol, and illicit substances, and those with friends who misuse alcohol and drugs tend to be more vulnerable to them. The influence of the Internet and social media in the development of risky behaviors is also concerning. Therefore, positive parenting and healthy friendships in adolescence are undisputable to reduce these behaviors. Dental providers also can play an important mentorship role for their young patients by being astute to potential problems, asking screening questions, explaining the negative effects of addictions in the oral cavity, and diagnosing oral lesions early to prevent progression to aggressive disease.

CLINICS CARE POINTS

- Understanding social determinants of health is a tenet of contemporary dental practice that cannot be ignored.
- The dental provider must ask questions about sensitive topics such as sexual behavior, use of drugs, alcohol, Internet addiction, driving safety, and so forth, to provide holistic care to young patients.
- Dental practitioners must familiarize themselves with local laws about adolescent rights to privacy and confidentiality.
- The deleterious effects of illicit substances, Internet addiction, and heavy gaming on the body and mind are well documented.
- They can also lead to oral manifestations in the form of cancers, periodontal disease, ulcerations, lesions, and bleeding.
- Adolescents who show risky behaviors are also more likely to be inattentive to oral hygiene practices, have heightened caries experience, and gaps in oral health care access.
- To alleviate xerostomia caused by illicit substances, many individuals use soft drinks or sports drinks more frequently, increasing their caries and dental erosion risk.
- The HPV vaccine has led to a 64% reduction in HPV prevalence in young women. Dental practitioners must discuss its long-term benefits with patients and parents.
- Risky behaviors may also expose young patients to a higher risk of contracting coronavirus.

DISCLOSURE

The authors have nothing to disclose.

REFERENCES

1. U.S. Department of Health and Human Services. Centers for Disease Control and Prevention, National Center for Chronic Disease Prevention and Health

Promotion, Office on Smoking and Health. The health consequences of smoking—50 years of progress: a report of the surgeon general, 2014. Available at: https://www.ncbi.nlm.nih.gov/books/NBK179276/pdf/Bookshelf_NBK179276.pdf. Accessed January 14, 2021.

2. U.S. Department of Health and Human Services. Centers for Disease Control and Prevention, National Center for Chronic Disease Prevention and Health Promotion, Office on Smoking and Health. Preventing tobacco use among youth and young adults: a report of the surgeon general, 2012. Available at: https://www.ncbi.nlm.nih.gov/books/NBK99237/pdf/Bookshelf_NBK99237.pdf. Accessed January 14, 2021.

3. Gentzke AS, Wang TW, Jamal A, et al. Tobacco product use among middle and high school students, United States, 2020. MMWR Morb Mortal Wkly Rep 2020;69:1881–8.

4. Gentzke AS, Creamer M, Cullen KA, et al. Vital signs: Tobacco product use among middle and high school students—United States, 2011–2018. MMWR Morb Mortal Wkly Rep 2019;68:157–64.

5. Wang TW, Gentzke AS, Creamer MR, et al. Tobacco product use and associated factors among middle and high school students – United States, 2019. MMWR Surveill Summ Rep 2019;68:1–22.

6. Wang TW, Gentzke A, Sharapova S, et al. Tobacco product use among middle and high school students – United States, 2011-2017. MMWR Morb Mortal Wkly Rep 2018;67(22):629–33.

7. U.S. Department of Health and Human Services. Reducing Tobacco Use: A Report of the Surgeon General. Atlanta, Georgia: U.S. Department of Health and Human Services, Centers for Disease Control and Prevention, National Center for Chronic Disease Prevention and Health Promotion, Office on Smoking and Health, 2000. Available at: https://www.cdc.gov/tobacco/data_statistics/sgr/2000/complete_report/pdfs/fullreport.pdf. Accessed January 28, 2021.

8. Centers for Disease Control and Prevention. Combustible and smokeless tobacco use among high school athletes — United States, 2001–2013. MMWR Morb Mortal Wkly Rep 2015;64(34):935–9.

9. National Institute on Drug Abuse. Research report series: Tobacco/Nicotine (NIH publication number 16-4342). Available at: https://d14rmgtrwzf5a.cloudfront.net/sites/default/files/tobaccorrs_1_2016.pdf. Accessed January 12, 2021.

10. Couch ET, Chaffee BW, Gansky SA, et al. The changing tobacco landscape: what dental professionals need to know. J Am Dent Assoc 2016;147:561–9.

11. Winn DM. Tobacco use and oral disease. J Dent Educ 2001;65:306–12.

12. Nicotine and health. Drug Ther Bull 2014;52(7):78–81.

13. Jones CM, Clayton HB, Deputy NP, et al. Prescription opioid misuse and use of alcohol and other substances among high school students - Youth Risk Behavior Survey, United States, 2019. MMWR Suppl 2020;69(Suppl 1):38–46.

14. Er V, Campbell R, Hickman M, et al. The relative importance of perceived substance misuse use by different peers on smoking, alcohol and illicit drug use in adolescence. Drug Alcohol Depend 2019;204:107464.

15. Degenhardt L, Hall W. Extent of illicit drug use and dependence, and their contribution to the global burden of disease. Lancet 2012;379:55–70.

16. Fergusson DM, Boden JM, Horwood LJ. Cannabis use and other illicit drug use: testing the cannabis gateway hypothesis. Addiction 2006;101:556–69.

17. Wong S-W, Lin H-C. Medical marijuana legalization and associated illicit drug use and prescription medication misuse among adolescents in the US. Addict Behav 2019;90:48–54.
18. Kulak JA, Griswold KS. Adolescent substance use and misuse: recognition and management. Am Fam Physician 2019;99:689–96.
19. Whiting PF, Wolff RF, Deshpande S, et al. Cannabinoids for medical use: a systematic review and meta-analysis. JAMA 2015;313:2456–73.
20. McGill N. As marijuana decriminalization spreads, public health prepares: health effects, regulations examined. Nation's Health 2014;44(7):1–14. Available at: https://www.thenationshealth.org/content/44/7/1.3. Accessed January 14, 2021.
21. Pacek LR, Mauro PM, Martins SS. Perceived risk of regular cannabis use in the United States from 2002 to 2012: differences by sex, age, and race/ethnicity. Drug Alcohol Depend 2015;149:232–44.
22. Jacobus J, Tapert SF. Effects of cannabis on the adolescent brain. Curr Pharm Des 2014;20:2186–93.
23. Broyd SJ, van Hell HH, Beale C, et al. Acute and chronic effects of cannabinoids on human cognition - a systematic review. Biol Psychiatry 2016;79:557–67.
24. Malone DT, Hill MN, Rubino T. Adolescent cannabis use and psychosis: epidemiology and neurodevelopmental models. Br J Pharmacol 2010;160:511–22.
25. Goyal H, Awad HH, Ghali JK. Role of cannabis in cardiovascular disorders. J Thorac Dis 2017;9(7):2079–92.
26. Rechthand MM, Bashirelahi N. What every dentist needs to know about cannabis. Gen Dent 2016;64:40–3.
27. Cho CM, Hirsch R, Johnstone S. General and oral health implications of cannabis use. Aust Dent J 2005;50:70–4.
28. Joshi S, Ashley M. Cannabis: a joint problem for patients and the dental profession. Br Dent J 2016;220:597–601.
29. Silk H, Kwok A. Addressing adolescent oral health: a review. Pediatr Rev 2017; 38:61–8.
30. Jager G, Witkamp RF. The endocannabinoid system and appetite: relevance for food reward. Nutr Res Rev 2014;27:172–85.
31. Versteeg PA, Slot DE, van der Velden U, et al. Effect of cannabis usage on the oral environment: a review. Int J Dent Hyg 2008;6:315–20.
32. Zhang Z-F, Morgenstern H, Spitz MR, et al. Marijuana use and increased risk of squamous cell carcinoma of the head and neck. Cancer Epidemiol Biomarkers Prev 1999;8:1071–8.
33. Chisini LA, Cademartori MG, Francia A, et al. Is the use of cannabis associated with periodontitis? A systematic review and meta-analysis. J Periodont Res 2019;54:311–7.
34. Thomson W, Poulton R, Broadbent JM, et al. Cannabis smoking and periodontal disease among young adults. JAMA 2008;299:525–31.
35. Duane B. Further evidence that periodontal bone loss increases with smoking and age. Evid Based Dent 2014;15:72–3.
36. Jamieson LM, Gunthorpe W, Cairney SJ, et al. Substance use and periodontal disease among Australian aboriginal young adults. Addiction 2010;105:719–26.
37. Maloney WJ, Raymond GF. Common substances and medications of abuse. In: O'Neil M, editor. The ADA practical guide to substance abuse disorders and safe prescribing. Hoboken, NJ: John Wiley & Sons, Inc.; 2015. p. 62–76.
38. Grafton SE, Huang PN, Vieira AR. Dental treatment planning considerations for patients using cannabis: a case report. J Am Dent Assoc 2016;147:354–61.

39. Hasan A, Sharma V. Substance abuse and conscious sedation: theoretical and practical considerations. Br Dent J 2019;227:923–7.

40. Beaulieu P. Anesthetic implications of recreational drug use. Can J Anesth 2017; 64:1236–64.

41. Maloney WJ, Raymond G. The significance of ecstasy use to dental practice. NY State Dent J 2014;80:24–7.

42. Antoniazzi RP, Sari AR, Casarin M, et al. Association between crack cocaine use and reduced salivary flow. Braz Oral Res 2017;31:e42.

43. Abebe W. Khat and synthetic cathinones: emerging drugs of abuse with dental implications. Oral Surg Oral Med Oral Pathol Oral Radiol 2018;125:140–6.

44. Hughes FJ, Bartold PM. Periodontal complications of prescription and recreational drugs. Periodontol 2000 2018;78:47–58.

45. Hegazi F, Alhazmi H, Abdullah A, et al. Prevalence of oral conditions among methamphetamine users: NHANES 2009-2014. J Public Health Dent 2021; 81:21–8.

46. Centers for Disease Control and Prevention, National Center for Injury Prevention and Control. Injury prevention and control, July 2020. Available at: https://www.cdc.gov/injury/wisqars/index.html. Accessed January 12, 2021.

47. Insurance Institute for Highway Safety. Fatality facts 2019 Teenagers. Available at: https://www.iihs.org/topics/fatality-statistics/detail/teenagers. Accessed January 12, 2021.

48. Ouimet MC, Pradhan AK, Brooks-Russell A, et al. Young drivers and their passengers: a systematic review of epidemiological studies on crash risk. J Adolesc Health 2015;57(1 Suppl):S24–35.

49. Gershon P, Ehsani JP, Zhu C, et al. Crash risk and risky driving behavior among adolescents during learner and independent driving periods. J Adolesc Health 2018;63:568–74.

50. Simons-Morton B, Lerner N, Singer J. The observed effects of teenage passengers on the risky driving behavior of teenage drivers. Accid Anal Prev 2005; 37(6):973–82.

51. Enriquez, J. (2019, August). Occupant restraint use in 2018: Results from the NOPUS controlled intersection study (Report No. DOT HS 812 781). Washington, DC: National Highway Traffic Safety Administration. Available at: https://crashstats.nhtsa.dot.gov/Api/Public/ViewPublication/812781. Accessed January 21, 2021.

52. Yellman MA, Bryan L, Sauber-Schatz EK, et al. Transportation risk behaviors among high school students — Youth Risk Behavior Survey, United States, 2019. MMWR Suppl 2020;69(Suppl-1):77–83.

53. National Highway Traffic Safety Administration. Traffic Safety Facts 2018 Data Speeding. (Report No. DOT HS 812 932). U.S. Department of Transportation; April 2020. Available at: https://crashstats.nhtsa.dot.gov/Api/Public/ViewPublication/812932. Accessed January 21, 2021.

54. Voas RB, Torres P, Romano E, et al. Alcohol-related risk of driver fatalities: an update using 2007 data. J Stud Alcohol Drugs 2012;73:341–50.

55. Torstveit MK, Rosenvinge JH, Sundgot-Borgen J. Prevalence of eating disorders and the predictive power of risk models in female elite athletes: a controlled study. Scand J Med Sci Sports 2008;18:108–18.

56. Agaku IT, Singh T, Jones SE, et al. Combustible and smokeless tobacco use among high school athletes—United States, 2001–2013. MMWR Morb Mortal Wkly Rep 2015;64:935–9.

57. Nicholls AR, Cope E, Bailey R, et al. Children's first experience of taking anabolic-androgenic steroids can occur before their 10th birthday: a systematic

review identifying 9 factors that predicted doping among young people. Front Psychol 2017;8:1015.

58. Williams GC, Burns KE, Batistta K, et al. High school sport participation and substance use: a cross-sectional analysis of students from the COMPASS study. Addict Behav Rep 2020;12:100298.

59. Milicic S, Pierard E, DeCicca P, et al. Examining the association between physical activity, sedentary behavior and sport participation with e-cigarette use and smoking status in a large sample of Canadian youth. Nicotine Tob Res 2019;21: 285–92.

60. Halstead ME, Walter KD. Sport-related concussion in children and adolescents. Pediatrics 2010;126:597–615.

61. Ranalli DN, Elderkin DL. Oral health issues for adolescent athletes. Dent Clin North Am 2006;50:119–37.

62. Ranalli DN. A sports dentistry trauma control plan for children and adolescents. J Southeast Soc Pediatr Dent 2002;8:8–9.

63. Tesini DA, Soporowski NJ. Epidemiology of orofacial sports-related injuries. Dent Clin North Am 2000;44:1–18.

64. Ranalli DN. Prevention of sport-related dental traumatic injuries. Dent Clin North Am 2000;44:19–33.

65. de Queiroz Gonçalves PH, Guimarães LS, de Azeredo FN, et al. Dental erosion prevalence and its relation to isotonic drinks in athletes: a systematic review and meta-analysis. Sport Sci Health 2020;16:207–16.

66. Buczkowska-Radlińska J, Łagocka R, Kaczmarek W, et al. Prevalence of dental erosion in adolescent competitive swimmers exposed to gas-chlorinated swimming pool water. Clin Oral Investig 2013;17:579–83.

67. Sartor CE, Jackson KM, McCutcheon VV, et al. Progression form first drink, first intoxication, and regular drinking to alcohol use disorder: a comparison of African American and European American youth. Alcohol Clin Exp Res 2016;40: 1515–23.

68. McCutcheon VV, Agrawal A, Kuo SI-C, et al. Associations of parental alcohol use disorders and parental separation with offspring initiation of alcohol, cigarette and cannabis and sexual debut in high-risk families. Addiction 2018;113: 336–45.

69. Anderson P, de Brujin A, Angus K, et al. Impact of alcohol advertising and media exposure on adolescent alcohol use: a systematic review of longitudinal studies. Alcohol Alcohol 2009;44:229–43.

70. Jones SA, Lueras JM, Nagel BJ. Effects of binge drinking on the developing brain. Alcohol Res 2018;39:87–96.

71. Yuen WS, Chan G, Bruno R, et al. Adolescent alcohol use trajectories: risk factors and adult outcomes. Pediatrics 2020;146:e20200440.

72. White HR, Stevens AK, Hayes K, et al. Changes in alcohol consumption among college students due to COVID-19: effects of campus closure and residential change. J Stud Alcohol Drugs 2020;81:725–30.

73. Skrypnikov AN, Sheshukova OV, Kazakov OA, et al. Oral status in adolescents with alcohol addiction. Wlad Lek 2019;72(5 cz2):970–1.

74. Maier H, Weidauer H, Zöller J, et al. Effect of chronic alcohol consumption on the morphology of the oral mucosa. Alcohol Clin Exp Res 1994;18:387–91.

75. Pulikkotil SJ, Nath S, Muthukumaraswamy LD, et al. Alcohol consumption is associated with periodontitis. A systematic review and meta-analysis of observational studies. Community Dent Health 2020;37:12–21.

76. Little JW, Miller CS, Rhodus NL. Drug and alcohol abuse. In: Little and Falace's dental management of the medically compromised patient. 9th edition. St. Louis: Elsevier; 2018. p. 581–5.

77. Freddo SL, da Cunha IP, Bulgareli JV, et al. Relations of drug use and socioeconomic factors with adherence to dental treatment among adolescents. BMC Oral Health 2018;18:221.

78. Oliveira Filho PM, Jorge KO, Ferreira EF, et al. Association between dental trauma and alcohol use among adolescents. Dent Traumatol 2013;29:372–7.

79. McAllister P, Laverick S, Makubate B, et al. Alcohol consumption and interpersonal injury in a pediatric oral and maxillofacial trauma population: a retrospective review of 1,192 trauma patients. Craniomaxillofac Trauma Reconstr 2015; 8:83–7.

80. Guo W, Tao Y, Li X, et al. Associations of internet addiction severity with psychopathology, serious mental illness, and suicidality: large-sample cross-sectional study. J Med Internet Res 2020;22:e17560.

81. Romer D, Bagdasarov Z, More E. Older versus new media and well-being of United States youth: results form a national longitudinal panel. J Adolesc Health 2013;52:613–9.

82. Marino C, Gini G, Vieno A, et al. The associations between problematic Facebook use, psychological distress and well-being among adolescents and young adults: a systematic review and meta-analysis. J Affect Disord 2018;226: 274–81.

83. Ho RC, Zhang MWB, Tsang TY, et al. The association between internet addiction and psychiatric co-morbidity: a meta-analysis. BMC Psychiatry 2014;14:183.

84. Petry NM, Rehbein F, Ko C-H, et al. Internet gaming disorder in the DSM-5. Curr Psychiatry Rep 2015;17(9):72.

85. Desai RA, Krishnan-Sarin S, Cavallo D, et al. Video-gaming among high school students: health correlates, gender differences, and problematic gaming. Pediatrics 2010;126:e1414–24.

86. Gentile D. Pathological video-game use among youth ages 8 to 18. A national study. Psychol Sci 2009;20(5):594–602.

87. Savolainen I, Kaakinen M, Sirola A, et al. Online relationships and social media interaction in youth problem gambling: a four-country study. Int J Environ Res Public Health 2020;17(21):8133.

88. Peters EN, Nordeck C, Zanetti G, et al. Relationship of gambling with tobacco, alcohol, and illicit drug use among adolescents in the USA: review of the literature 2000-2014. Am J Addict 2015;24:206–16.

89. Hollen L, Dorner R, Griffiths MD, et al. Gambling in young adults aged 17-24 years: a population-based study. J Gambl Stud 2020;36:747–66.

90. Wardle H, McManus S. Suicidality and gambling among young adults in Great Britain: results from a cross-sectional online survey. Lancet Public Health 2021; 6:e39–49.

91. Pisarska A, Ostaszewski K. Factors associated with youth gambling: longitudinal study among high school students. Public Health 2020;184:33–40.

92. Henkel D, Zemlin U. Social inequity and substance use and problematic gambling among adolescents and young adults: a review of epidemiological surveys in Germany. Curr Drug Abuse Rev 2016;9:26–48.

93. Petruzelka B, Vacek J, Gavurova B, et al. Interaction of socioeconomic status with risky internet use, gambling and substance use in adolescents from a structurally disadvantaged region in Central Europe. Int J Environ Res Public Health 2020;17:4803.

94. US National Human Trafficking Hotline, 2019 data report. Available at: https:// humantraffickinghotline.org/. Accessed January 19, 2021.

95. US Department of Justice. Child sex trafficking. Available at: justice.gov/ criminal-ceos/child-sex-trafficking. Accessed January 11, 2021.

96. Institute of Medicine and National Research Council of the National Academies, Committee on the Commercial Sexual Exploitation and Sex Trafficking of Minors in the United States, Board of Children, Youth and Families. In: Clayton EW, Krugman RD, Simon P, editors. Confronting commercial sexual exploitation and sex trafficking of minors in the United States. Washington, DC: The National Academies Press; 2013. p. 271–96. Available at: https://ojjdp.ojp.gov/sites/g/ files/xyckuh176/files/pubs/243838.pdf. Accessed January 11, 2021.

97. Fedina L, Williamson C, Perdue T. Risk factors for domestic child sex trafficking in the United States. J Interpers Violence 2019;34:2653–73.

98. Baldwin SB, Eisenman DP, Sayles JN, et al. Identification of human trafficking victims in health care settings. Health Hum Rights 2011;13:E36–49.

99. Chaffee T, English A. Sex trafficking of adolescents and young adults in the United States: healthcare provider's role. Curr Opin Obstet Gynecol 2015;27: 339–44.

100. O'Callaghan MG. Human trafficking and the dental professional. J Am Dent Assoc 2012;143:498–504.

101. US Department of State. Trafficking in persons report. 20th edition. Washington, DC: US Department of State Publication; 2020. p. 30. Available at: https://www. state.gov/wp-content/uploads/2020/06/2020-TIP-Report-Complete-062420-FINAL.pdf. Accessed January 19, 2021.

102. Martinez GM, Abma JC. Sexual activity and contraceptive use among teenagers aged 15-19 in the United States, 2015-2017. US Department of Health and Human Services, Centers for Disease Control and Prevention. NHCS Data Brief No. 366, May 2020. Available at: https://www.cdc.gov/nchs/data/databriefs/db366-h.pdf. Accessed February 15, 2021.

103. Abma JC, Martinez GM. Sexual activity and contraceptive use among teenagers in the United States, 2011-2015. US Department of Health and Human Services, Centers for Disease Control and Prevention. National Health Statistics Reports N0. 104, June 22, 2017. Data Brief No. 366, May 2020. Available at: https:// www.cdc.gov/nchs/data/nhsr/nhsr104.pdf. Accessed February 15, 2021.

104. Scott RH, Wellings K, Lindberg L. Adolescent sexual acitivity, contraceptive use, and pregnancy in Britain and the U.S.: A multidecade comparison. J Adolesc Health 2020;66:582–8.

105. Shannon CL, Klausner JD. The growing epidemic of sexually transmitted infections in adolescents: a neglected population. Curr Opin Pediatr 2018;30: 137–43.

106. Centers for Disease Control and Prevention. STDs in adolescents and young adults. Sexually Transmitted Diseases Surveillance; 2018. Available at: https:// www.cdc.gov/std/stats18/adolescents.htm. Accessed February 15, 2021.

107. Prinstein MJ, Meade CS, Cohen GL. Adolescent oral sex, peer popularity, and perceptions of best friends' sexual behavior. J Pediatr Psychol 2003;28:243–9.

108. National Academies of Sciences, Engineering, and Medicine; Health and Medicine Division; Division of Behavioral and Social Sciences and Education; Board of Children, Youth and Families; Committee on Applying Lessons of Optimal Adolescent Health to Improve Behavioral Outcomes for Youth. In: Kahn NF, Graham R, editors. Promoting positive adolescent health behaviors and outcomes: thriving in the 21st century. Washington, DC: National Academies Press;

2020. p. 79–88. Available at: https://www.ncbi.nlm.nih.gov/books/NBK554992/pdf/Bookshelf_NBK554992.pdf. Accessed February 16, 2021.

109. Lindberg LD, Santelli JS, Desai S. Changing patterns of contraceptive use and the decline in rates of pregnancy and birth among US adolescents, 2007-2014. J Adolesc Health 2018;63:253–6.

110. Bruce A, Rogers R III. Oral manifestations of sexually transmitted diseases. Clin Dermatol 2004;22:520–7.

111. Centers for Division Control and Prevention, Sexually Transmitted Diseases (STDs). STD risk and oral sex – CDC fact sheet. Available at: https://www.cdc.gov/std/healthcomm/stdfact-stdriskandoralsex.htm. Accessed January 14, 2021.

112. Seibt CE, Munerato MC. Secondary syphilis in the oral cavity and the role of the dental surgeon in STD prevention, diagnosis and treatment: a case series study. Braz J Infect Dis 2016;20:393–8.

Eating Disorders in the Adolescent Patient

Dennis N. Ranalli, DDS, MDS[a,b], Deborah Studen-Pavlovich, DMD[a,*]

KEYWORDS

- Adolescent • Eating disorders • Systemic manifestations • Oral sequelae
- Dental intervention

KEY POINTS

- The adolescent period is one in which individuals frequently engage in eating patterns that may negatively impact their overall well-being and dental health.
- Dental practitioners have a responsibility to recognize their adolescent patients who fulfill specific criteria for various eating disorders.
- Dental practitioners require foundational knowledge concerning the epidemiology and systemic effects of anorexia nervosa, female athlete triad, bulimia nervosa, obesity, and binge eating.
- Dental practitioners should possess the discernment to refer patients with eating disorders to other appropriate medical, psychological, and nutritional specialists.
- Dental practitioners must be proficient to assess intraoral manifestations of adolescent eating disorders and provide proper dental treatment or appropriate referral.

INTRODUCTION

Proper diet and nutrition are key components that contribute to steady growth and development during the adolescent period. Unfortunately there are many adolescents and young adults who engage in eating behaviors that interfere with their overall health and well-being, including oral and dental health.

It is important at the outset to distinguish between 2 terms that relate to aberrant adolescent eating behaviors, namely, *eating disorders* and *disordered eating*. *Disordered eating* represents a range of multidimensional non-normative eating behaviors that may include practices such as fad diets, fasting, vomiting, misuse of diet pills, diuretics, or laxatives. In contrast, the term *eating disorders* represents patterns of malnutrition with inherent life-threatening potential that stem from underlying and complex psychiatric illnesses.[1]

a Department of Pediatric Dentistry, University of Pittsburgh School of Dental Medicine, 3501 Terrace Street, Pittsburgh, PA 15261, USA; b Sports Medicine and Nutrition, School of Health and Rehabilitation Sciences, University of Pittsburgh, Pittsburgh, PA, USA
* Corresponding author.
E-mail address: das12@pitt.edu

Dent Clin N Am 65 (2021) 689–703
https://doi.org/10.1016/j.cden.2021.06.009
dental.theclinics.com

For this article, our scope will be confined to the categories of eating disorders as follows: (1) underweight and wasting patterns of malnutrition (*anorexia nervosa* [AN], and the *female athlete triad*); (2) underweight and/or normal weight patterns of malnutrition (*bulimia nervosa* [BN]); (3) overweight patterns of malnutrition (*obesity*, and *binge eating*).

As of this writing, the world is in the midst of the COVID-19 pandemic. Dental professionals daily must confront the various aspects of this disease as well as ongoing updates regarding mitigation protocols.[2] Although the long-term effects of the COVID-19 pandemic on adolescents with eating disorders and obesity have yet to be documented definitively, early research findings have been revealing. Where appropriate, these findings are included in the text.

Our intent for this article is to provide practicing dental professionals with current scientific evidence on adolescent eating disorders and obesity that may influence dentofacial development and intraoral conditions that require therapeutic dental interventions.

UNDERWEIGHT AND WASTING PATTERNS OF MALNUTRITION
Anorexia Nervosa

As we begin to explore the various patterns of eating disorders among adolescents, the term *anorexia* is likely to be among the most familiar. It is important to note, however, that *anorexia* is sometimes mistakenly used as a synonym for AN. *Anorexia* (*without appetite*) is defined simply as a loss of appetite or an inability to eat. Loss of appetite may be a secondary manifestation of other conditions such as depression, infection, cancer, or the side effects of medication, among others.[3] From a dental perspective, for example, some adolescent patients may experience a temporary loss of appetite after extraction of third molars.

In contradistinction, the term *Anorexia Nervosa* (*nervous loss of appetite*) represents a complex psychological disorder with the potential to become life-threatening. This eating disorder consists of limiting food consumption to an extreme to maintain an abnormally low body weight, accompanied by cognitive distortions regarding body image. There are 2 clinical subtypes of *AN*, food restricting and food purging. It should be pointed out that terms used previously such as "self-inflicted" starvation or a "refusal" to maintain body weight implied a willfulness on the part of the patient. Current thinking now focuses more attention on behaviors such as "restricting calorie intake."[1,3,4]

Epidemiology, prevalence, demographics

The onset of *AN* commonly occurs during the adolescent period with a peak range between 15 and 19 years of age. In the United States (US) and Europe, lifetime prevalence of *AN* is relatively low between 0.3% and 0.5%. While the prevalence for males and females may have increased somewhat over time, late adolescent and young adult females continue to account for 90% of reported cases. Although usually thought of as a disease primarily associated with white, middle-class females, there have been some increases in the frequency of *AN* noted in both minority populations and among those in lower socioeconomic strata.[4] *AN* is associated often with various psychiatric comorbidities such as major depression, anxiety disorders, obsessive-compulsive disorder (OCD), as well as substance abuse.

Serious confounding factors of current relevance are health concerns surrounding the COVID-19 pandemic. As a novel coronavirus appeared then spread rapidly during 2020 resulting in the worldwide COVID-19 pandemic, concerns regarding the implications of this disease on global behaviors and health conditions expanded at a pace commensurate with the spread of the disease. While the total impact has yet to be determined fully, preliminary studies regarding the pandemic's influence on the epidemiology, prevalence, and demographics of AN suggest an increase in both the number and severity of cases.[5]

Diagnostic criteria

The criteria for a diagnosis of AN are established by the American Psychiatric Association; the most recent iteration being 2013. This revision (Diagnostic and Statistical Manual of Mental Disorders, fifth Edition [DSM-5])[6] contains some changes differing from those in the previous version (DSM-4).[7]

To establish a diagnosis of AN, the patient must meet all the current criteria (DSM-5):[6]

- Restricted food intake with weight loss or a failure to gain weight. A "significantly low body weight" greater than what would be expected for peers of the same age, sex, and height.
- Fear of gaining weight or becoming fat
- Distorted self-image or an unrealistic view of their condition (denial)

There were 2 changes in the diagnostic criteria between the previous (DSM-4)[7] and the current iterations (DSM-5)[6]:

- *Amenorrhea* was eliminated. The rationale behind this change was twofold: (1) It allows males to meet the criteria; (2) it allows females to meet the criteria who continue to menstruate despite extreme weight loss and malnutrition.
- The low weight criterion was revised to allow more subjectivity and clinical judgment enabling professionals to integrate a patient's unique growth trajectory and weight history into the overall assessment.

Systemic effects

While it is not within the purview of the dental profession to diagnose or to treat the array of medical or psychological conditions that patients with AN may demonstrate, it is, nonetheless, essential for dentists to be sufficiently knowledgeable to recognize the signs and symptoms of this eating disorder and to initiate appropriate referrals as needed.

Physical signs. While some patients with AN may intentionally fail to report the existence of their eating disorder, others may even deny the existence of such a problem. Visual observation by the dental team can be invaluable in recognizing an adolescent with AN. The physical signs and symptoms that may be observable in the dental environment begin with the recognition that such patients are apt to appear along a range of body forms from slim to emaciated. Dehydration may be apparent, for example, the patient's skin may appear dry or exhibit a yellowish cast. Fingernails may appear brittle, and nail beds may have a bluish discoloration. Fine lanugo body hair may be present, but scalp hair may be thinning, and some patients may admit to spontaneous hair loss. The eyes may appear sunken with dark shadows. Patients suffering from AN may complain of fatigue, insomnia, dizziness, fainting, or intolerance to cold.[1,3,4]

Medical complications. Serious systemic manifestations have been reported for individuals with AN. If malnutrition becomes chronic and severe, every organ has the potential to suffer damage to the extent that it may reach a level that is not fully reversible. Death becomes a possibility.[1,3,4]

Medical complications may include, but are not limited to, the following systems[1,3,4]:

- Cardiovascular: hypotension, syncope, bradycardia, mitral valve prolapse, heart failure
- Gastrointestinal: bloating, constipation, nausea, vomiting
- Hematopoietic: anemia, thrombocytopenia
- Reproductive: females, absence of a period; males, decreased testosterone
- Musculoskeletal: muscle loss, *osteoporosis*, elevated fracture risk
- Metabolic: low blood levels of potassium, sodium, or chloride; metabolic alkalosis

Psychological disorders. In addition to the many physical signs and medical complications described, *AN* may be associated with a wide range of psychiatric comorbidities such as major depression, anxiety and other mood disorders, personality disorders, OCD, as well as alcohol and substance abuse. There may be an increased tendency for self-injury, suicidal thoughts, or suicide attempts. It is important to note that the mortality rate associated with *AN* is believed to be the highest among psychiatric illnesses.[1,3,4] Research findings in behavioral genetics including family, twin, and molecular genetic studies suggest that substantial genetic influences might contribute to underlying causes of eating disorders.[8]

Intraoral hard- and soft-tissue effects

Considering the multiplicity of factors that may coexist in patients with *AN*, it should not be surprising that these patients may exhibit a wide range of oral and dental conditions.[9] The misuse of fad diets, diet pills, diuretics, or laxatives can have negative impact on the oral cavity in the form of *xerostomia*. Less than normal salivary flow interferes with the normal self-cleansing of the hard and soft tissues of the mouth. This dry type of environment fosters the development of dental caries.

Dehydration and xerostomia also may affect the soft tissues of the mouth. The lips may be dry and chapped; the corners of the mouth may develop angular cheilitis. Intraorally, the gingiva may look pale, or gingivitis with bleeding may be present. The palate may have the look of yellow-orange discoloration, and there may be signs of palatal petechiae. Atrophic mucosa may be observable.[9,10]

Patients with the clinical subtype of *chronic purging AN* may exhibit swelling of the parotid glands (*sialadenosis*) and are at increased risk for the development of a specific type of enamel erosion of the lingual surfaces of the teeth (*perimylolysis*)[9,10] (**Fig. 1**). As lingual erosion progresses over time from repeated episodes of acidic vomitus, chipping of the incisal edges of the anterior teeth begins to occur. That coupled with the occlusal erosion of the posterior teeth may lead to a loss in vertical dimension (**Fig. 2**) and restorations that appear above the occlusal surfaces (**Fig. 3**) which can contribute to the development of temporomandibular joint symptoms.[11]

In addition to temporomandibular symptoms brought on by the loss of vertical dimension from *perimylolysis*, other psychiatric comorbidities such as major depression, anxiety disorders, or OCD may contribute to the clenching or grinding of teeth, placing added stresses on the joint and muscles. The symptoms of *temporomandibular disorder* may include dizziness, headaches, facial pain, and muscle fatigue.[11]

For those individuals with *AN* whose condition progresses to chronic *amenorrhea*, osteopenia and premature osteoporosis may develop. This bone loss may be linked to a loss of alveolar bone.[12]

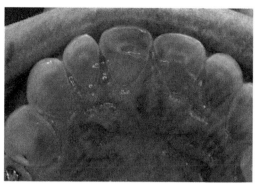

Fig. 1. Lingual view illustrating perimylolysis with dentin exposure on all lingual surfaces of the maxillary anterior teeth in this 25-year-old patient recovering from chronic purging anorexia nervosa. (*Courtesy of* Dr. Keith Alpine, prosthodontist.)

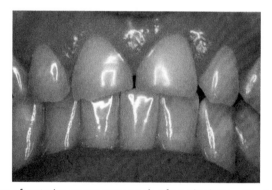

Fig. 2. Labial view of anterior permanent teeth after gingivectomies to increase clinical crown lengths in the same patient. (*Courtesy of* Dr. Keith Alpine, prosthodontist.)

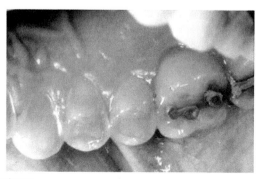

Fig. 3. Floating amalgam.

UNDERWEIGHT AND WASTING PATTERNS OF MALNUTRITION
Female Athlete Triad

The term *female athlete triad* was first introduced in 1992 by the American College of Sports Medicine.[13] It was a term used to describe a clinical pattern observed among adolescent and young adult female athletes in sports such as gymnastics and figure skating, among others. Body image in these competitive sports contributes to the esthetic effect of the athletic performance. The same may be said for ballet dancers whose artistic performances are enhanced by their athleticism.

The *female athlete triad* shares characteristics similar to those found in nonathlete patients with *AN*; namely a complex psychological eating disorder that limits food consumption to an extreme. That coupled with high-intensity athletic training regimens may result in *amenorrhea* and *osteoporosis*.[11,14] However, based on a revised position statement that was issued by the American College of Sports Medicine in 2007, the criteria for establishing a definitive diagnosis of the *female athlete triad* have been modified.[15,16]

In this more recent iteration, the triad is currently characterized as a spectrum of interrelated conditions and complications. These include 3 components that were renamed: *menstrual function*, *low energy availability* with or without eating disorder, and *low bone mineral density*. According to this definition, athletes may present with any of the triad components, and they need not be present simultaneously for that individual athlete to suffer negative health consequences.[13,14,16]

Based on this latest clarification of the *female athlete triad* spectrum, the prevalence for patients demonstrating simultaneously all 3 of the components ranges from 1% to 2% among high school–aged girls and 0% to 16% for all female athletes.[17,18] Prevalence of 2 concurrent components ranges from 4% to 18%, and for a single component, 16% to 54% in high school–aged female athletes.[17–22]

The systemic effects as well as the intraoral hard- and soft-tissue findings for the *female athlete triad* are essentially the same as those described in the section under *AN*.

UNDERWEIGHT AND/OR NORMAL WEIGHT PATTERNS OF MALNUTRITION
Bulimia Nervosa

Another potentially life-threatening eating disorder named *bulimia nervosa* became recognized in the 1970s[23] and was later identified as a specific disorder in the 1980s to establish the distinction between symptoms of *bulimia* (binge eating) and the *binge eating/purge syndrome*.[24] Patients with *BN*, particularly the purging type, share similar signs and symptoms as those with *AN*. The essential difference between these 2 eating disorders relates to body weight of the individual. Those with *BN* may be of normal or above-normal weight, whereas individuals with *AN* continue to exhibit significant weight loss.

The binge-purge cycle involves eating large amounts of food followed by self-induced vomiting as one means of compensating for overindulgence. While patients with *AN* continue to severely lose weight over time, the physical effects of *BN* are manifested more in esophageal deterioration, menstrual irregularities, dental caries, perimylolysis, and vitamin deficiencies.

Epidemiology, prevalence, demographics

BN commonly begins in adolescence or early adulthood; onset before puberty or after the age of 40 years is uncommon.[6] Frequently, the binge eating begins during or shortly after an episode of dieting to lose weight; for others, the onset of *BN* may be precipitated by a stressful life event.

In the US, the lifetime prevalence of *BN* is 1.5% in females and 0.5% in males. The disorder occurs across gender, ethnicity, and socioeconomic strata with similar prevalence.[6] *BN* peaks in late adolescence and early adulthood in females; however, less is known about the prevalence in males because it is far less common than in females, with an approximately 10:1 female-to-male ratio.[6] *BN* occurs with similar frequencies in most industrialized countries, such as Canada, Australia, Japan, and many European countries.[6]

Diagnostic criteria

Three essential features must be present for a diagnosis of *BN*:

- Recurrent episodes of binge eating
- Recurrent inappropriate compensatory behaviors to prevent weight gain, such as self-induced vomiting, misuse of laxatives or diuretics
- The binge eating and inappropriate compensatory behavior both occur, on average, at least once a week for 3 months.[6]

While the severity of *AN* is graded based on body mass index (BMI), the severity of *BN* is based on the number of purging episodes during a given week. Degrees of severity are defined as follows:

- Mild, 1 to 3 episodes per week
- Moderate, 4 to 7 episodes per week
- Severe, 8 to 13 episodes per week
- Extreme, 14 or more episodes per week[6]

Individuals with *BN* usually are within normal weight or overweight ranges with BMIs of 18.5 to 30 in adults. For adolescents up to the age of 19 years, BMI is calculated as sex- and age-specific. The disorder may occur among obese individuals but is uncommon.

After binge eating, the most common compensatory method used among those with *BN* is self-induced vomiting. This technique along with the misuse of laxatives accounts for more than 90% of the purging behaviors in *BN*.[25]

Systemic effects

Medical conditions that are observed in *BN* primarily are associated with purging behaviors and may present themselves in a variety of ways including during physical examination and through abnormal laboratory test results.[25]

One specific dermatologic indicator that may appear is callous formation on the dorsal aspect of the finger or fingers used to self-induce vomiting. This finding is referred to Russell's sign and is the result of repetitive trauma and skin abrasions over time attempting to induce emesis.[23]

Self-induced vomiting also may result in subconjunctival hemorrhage and recurrent bouts of epistaxis.[24] Red patches in the white portions of the eyes may appear disfiguring but are benign. They may be observed by the dental professional during a recall examination and should prompt inquiry about how it may have occurred. Frequent nose bleeds also should prompt further questioning.

Patients who self-induce vomiting often will complain of symptoms similar to those reported with gastroesophageal reflux disease.[26] With repetitive vomiting, the esophageal musculature and epithelium are exposed to excessive acidic gastric contents and microtrauma. Consequences that may develop include esophagitis, esophageal erosions and ulcers, Barrett's esophagus, and bleeding.

Abnormalities in electrolyte test results may indicate such conditions as metabolic alkalosis and hypokalemia from repetitive purging. Ultimately, this may lead to dehydration.[25] Patients with *BN* may complain of dizziness, excessive thirst, and syncope. Cardiovascular and renal failure may occur in severe cases.

Similar to *AN*, *BN* is associated with various medical sequelae that depend primarily on the mode and frequency of purging. Some of these complications may be very serious, causing long-term or permanent damage to the adolescent.

Oral health effects

While examining the oral cavity, the dental professional may be the first health care provider to notice the effects of long-term, self-induced vomiting. Several abnormalities in the oral cavity have been reported and include

- Perimylolysis
- Reduced salivary flow rate
- Dental hypersensitivity
- Dental caries
- Sialadenosis
- Periodontal disease
- Xerostomia.[27]

The maxillary anterior teeth are affected most severely by repeated self-induced vomiting. Perimylolysis may appear as early as 6 months after the onset of purging.[27] The severity of this type of erosion is determined by the duration and frequency of vomiting, types of food eaten, oral hygiene, and the baseline quality of the tooth structure.[28] Although mandibular teeth may be affected, they are generally protected from gastric acid exposure by the tongue.[28]

An increased rate of dental caries may occur as a consequence of bingeing on large amounts of carbohydrates, poor oral hygiene, and increased intake of carbonated beverages, as well as acid exposure from purging.[27] Gingivitis and periodontal disease may result from repeated exposure to gastric acid. The gastric acid, in turn, may cause chronic gingival irritation and bleeding.

Sialadenosis, hypertrophy of the salivary glands, is a common occurrence, having been reported in 10% to 50% of patients with self-induced vomiting.[27] It generally appears bilaterally and only is minimally tender. The parotid glands are the most commonly affected salivary glands and often give patients "chipmunk-type" facies. It generally occurs 3 to 4 days after self-induced vomiting and may result from elevated serum amylase levels.[29]

OVERWEIGHT PATTERNS OF MALNUTRITION
Obesity

Obesity is a major, chronic health concern both globally and in the US. It continues to be the most prevalent nutritional disorder among children and adolescents, placing them at potential risk for a lifetime of poor health.[30] For the purposes of this article, we propose the notion of obesity as a continuum that may transcend childhood onto adolescence, young adulthood, and beyond. Unless the continuum is interrupted, the adverse effects continue to mount. For example, too little physical activity and too many calories from food and drinks are the main contributors to childhood obesity, but genetic and hormonal factors may play a role, as well. Childhood obesity may lead to psychological problems such as poor self-esteem and depression. Adolescents who are obese may develop hypertension, hypercholesterolemia, impaired glucose tolerance, and other systemic disorders. So, suffice it to say obesity is a major public health concern and a multifactorial disease with physical, psychological, and social consequences throughout the lifespan.

Epidemiology, prevalence, and demographics
The prevalence of obesity among children and adolescents has almost tripled since 2000. Currently, obesity affects 19.3% of all children and adolescents (14.4 million) aged 2 through 19 years in the US.[30] Americans, unfortunately, have one of the highest percentages of overweight adolescents among developed countries, and the probability of adolescent obesity persisting into adulthood is 80%.[30] Over the past 30 years, the rate of childhood obesity has more than doubled, and the rate of adolescent obesity has quadrupled.

Although the demand for nutrients during adolescence is greater because of physical growth and pubertal development, this period is associated with an increased risk for the development of obesity, especially for female teens who have a larger deposition of fat than muscle. Boys and girls differ in body composition, hormones, patterns of weight gain, and susceptibility to various social, ethnic, genetic, and environmental factors.[31]

Diagnostic criteria
Obesity for the childhood-adolescent continuum is defined as a BMI at or above the 95th percentile of the sex-specific BMI-for-age growth charts. In contrast, adult BMI does not depend on sex or age. The BMI is a noninvasive and indirect way of measuring body fat and is calculated by taking a person's weight (pounds) and dividing it by their height (inches) squared. It is not a diagnostic tool, but rather an assessment to screen for potential weight-related issues. In addition, because BMI charts were developed from a nationally representative population, as Americans become heavier, the sensitivity of this measurement decreases.[32] The American Academy of Pediatrics recommends using BMI as a screening tool for obesity in children starting at 2 years of age.[33] Oral health care professionals have ideal opportunities to intervene during routine recall examinations by measuring the patient's height and weight, followed by determining the patient's BMI. In addition, taking the patient's blood pressure may be an additional parameter related to obesity. If the BMI is in the overweight (85th to 95th percentile)/obese range and blood pressure in the hypertensive range, referral can be made to the patient's physician for follow-up care.

Systemic effects
The health consequences of obesity can present during the childhood-adolescent continuum, but the longer a person remains obese, the more that individual is at risk for health problems during adulthood. A high BMI during adolescence increases adult-onset diabetes and coronary artery diseases, threefold and fivefold, respectively.[34] One of the most serious comorbidities of childhood obesity is type 2 diabetes. Other comorbid conditions which may manifest as a result of childhood obesity include, but are not limited to,

- Hypertension
- Abnormal lipid profiles
- Nonalcoholic fatty live disease
- Gallstones
- Gastroesophageal reflux
- Polycystic ovary syndrome
- Obstructive sleep apnea
- Asthma
- Bone and joint problems.[35]

In addition, underlying psychiatric disorders, such as depression, poor self-esteem, anxiety, poor quality of life, and binge eating disorder, may cause or be a result of obesity.[36]

Binge eating disorder

Binge eating disorder, which occurs in approximately 20% to 40% of obese adolescents and adults, is one of the most recent eating disorders recognized in the DSM-5.[6] The disorder is characterized by recurrent episodes of eating large quantities of food, sometimes very quickly and to the point of becoming uncomfortable. In the binge eating disorder, the person does not use compensatory mechanisms such as purging to counteract the bingeing. The episode of binge eating must be characterized by both of the following:

- Eating, in a discrete period of time, an amount of food that is larger than what most people would eat in a similar period under similar circumstances and
- A sense of lack of control over eating during the episode.

Currently, it is the most common eating disorder in the US, three times more common than *AN* and *BN* combined.[37]

Oral health effects

Research related to the association between obesity and oral health has been reported in the literature related to dental caries, dental development, periodontal diseases, and sedation.[38–55] However, obesity is a multifactorial disease for which cause-and-effect relationships are difficult to establish definitively. Here, we focus on the following topics:

Dental caries

Similar to obesity, dental caries is a chronic, prevalent, multifactorial disease afflicting US children and adolescents. Dental caries and obesity both share one distinct contributing factor—diet; both of these conditions often are left untreated. In addition, dental caries is highly associated with lower socioeconomic status. Even though research on the association between obesity and dental caries has been conducted for many years, the results have been ambiguous.

In a recent systematic review of BMI and dental caries in subjects younger than 18 years, evidence of an association between BMI and caries was inconsistent.[38] Of the 4208 identified studies, this review included 84 that met the inclusion criteria for determining potential associations between BMI and caries:

- 26 studies showed a positive relationship
- 19 showed a negative association
- 43 found no association between the variables.[38]

Well-designed, longitudinal studies evaluating the association of various indicators of obesity and dental caries during childhood and adolescence may assist in elucidating this complex relationship.

Dental development

The biological processes of dental and skeletal development have been used as stable benchmarks to determine physical maturation.[40] Obese children have been shown to grow at an accelerated rate and reach skeletal maturity and puberty earlier,[41] and increased BMI has been associated with accelerated growth, premature puberty, and early sexual development.[42]

In numerous studies from various locations in the US, childhood obesity was found to be associated with accelerated dental development and eruption of permanent teeth, and patients with higher BMI values were more likely to have advanced dental development for their age at a significant level ($P<.001$).[43–45]

Other studies among various racial and ethnic groups (Hispanic, Asian, White, Black) demonstrated further that differences in dental age, when compared to chronologic age, were significantly greater in children who were overweight/obese versus their underweight/average counterparts.[43,44]

As the prevalence of obesity increases in the US, dental professionals need a better understanding of how obesity with increased BMI affects dental development. Predicting the stage of dental development, eruption and sequence in the mixed dentition are critical for appropriately timing dental treatments for best outcomes such as space maintenance by the pediatric dentist. The timing of orthodontic intervention based on dental age rather than chronologic age should be essential to the orthodontist in obtaining not only radiographic records but also BMI values. These same factors are key in evaluating adolescent prosthodontic patients for placement of an esthetic anterior implant based on both the dental and skeletal ages of the individual. For oral and maxillofacial surgeons, the timing of third molar extractions may be earlier for their obese adolescent patients than for nonobese and underweight patients.

Periodontal disease

An association between obesity and periodontal disease was first reported in 1998 in Japan.[46] Since then, a number of studies have identified obesity as a risk factor for the development of periodontal disease,[47–49] and several cross-sectional studies have reported that obesity is associated with increased prevalence of chronic periodontitis in adults.[50,51]

To better comprehend how obesity may contribute to periodontal disease, an understanding of how adipose tissue functions in the body is relevant. It is important to stress that adipose tissue is not merely a passive triglyceride reservoir of the body, but rather it generates vast amounts of cytokines and hormones, collectively called adipokines or adipocytokines.[52] These substances are involved in inflammatory processes that point toward similar pathways associated with the pathophysiology of obesity, periodontitis, and other related inflammatory diseases.[53] While the underlying biological mechanisms linking obesity with periodontitis are not fully understood, adipokines or adipocytokines may play a key role.

Associations between obesity and periodontal risk indicators in obese adolescents have been reported.[48] Given the generally high prevalence of obesity among adolescents globally, it seems prudent to investigate early markers of periodontal disease to better manage them. In a Belgian study of obese adolescents, the obese group showed higher incidence of caries, gingivitis, and plaque, although after adjusting for age and sex, obesity was associated significantly only with the presence of dental plaque ($P\leq.001$).[54] The obese participants reported a significantly elevated intake of sugar-rich and high caloric food than the normal weight group, a factor that may be contributory to the presence of dental plaque (**Fig. 4**).

In a Swedish study of obese and normal weight adolescents between the ages of 11 and 17.9 years, an association between obesity and periodontal risk indicators such as gingival inflammation, periodontal pocket depth, calculus, and incipient alveolar bone loss was demonstrated in the obese subjects.[48] These results further strengthen the potential negative impact of obesity on adolescent periodontal health.

Other studies evaluated the microbiome of obese adolescents in comparison to normal weight adolescents.[55] Obese subjects were found to harbor more periodontal

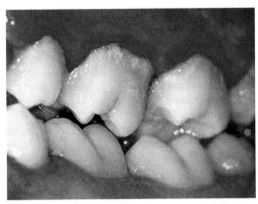

Fig. 4. Morbidly obese patient with copious deposits of plaque and calculus on buccal surfaces of maxillary posterior teeth. Note the fiery red nature of the gingival tissues.

pathogens such as *Veillonella*, *Haemophilus*, and *Prevotella* species than their normal weight counterparts. This distinct salivary microbiota may bring new insights into the etiology and prevention of periodontal disease in adolescents. It also highlights the importance of a close collaboration between dentists and pediatricians in the prevention and treatment of obesity.

In recognizing the periodontal implications associated with obesity, dental professionals should integrate BMI calculations as well as blood pressure readings as part of the assessment for their adolescent patients along with evaluating medical history risk factors. Initiating a dialog with the adolescent patient regarding obesity-related concerns can promote awareness for disease prevention.

Sedation/anesthesia
Obese adolescent patients who require the use of sedation or general anesthesia for dental treatment may exhibit physiologic changes as well as comorbidities that require evaluation by an anesthesiologist.[39] A detailed description is provided in the Matthew Cooke and Thomas Tanbonliong's article, "Sedation and Anesthesia for the Adolescent Dental Patient," in this issue.

Dental Recommendations
Throughout this article, our focus has been on nutrition as the key component that contributes to steady growth and development during the adolescent period and the negative consequences eating disorders exert on overall health and well-being, including oral and dental health of adolescent dental patients. The treatment of adolescents with eating disorders is often multifaceted and complex, requiring referrals not only to dental specialists but also to medical, psychological, and nutritional experts.

In our descriptions of each eating disorder including *AN*, *female athlete triad*, *BN*, obesity, and binge eating, we provided specifics of the oral and dental signs and symptoms that may be encountered in the day-to-day practice of general dentistry or in the specialty practices of pediatric dentistry, orthodontics and dentofacial orthopedics, periodontics, prosthodontics, and anesthesiology.

But regardless of the eating disorder exhibited by the adolescent, the essential first phase is to initiate a meticulous dental home care regimen. The basics of brushing and flossing cannot be overemphasized. For patients with xerostomia, oral rinses or salivary substitutes may be beneficial; for others, custom fluoride trays may mitigate caries activity or a nightguard for bruxism may alleviate muscle soreness.

Phase 2 includes scheduling more frequent recall appointments. This routine enables the dentist to better monitor patient compliance and to provide professional services such as prophylaxis, scaling, topical fluoride applications, and pit and fissure sealants. More frequent oral examinations provide the opportunity to discover hard- and soft-tissue changes at earlier stages and to initiate more conservative dental therapy. The assessment of adolescent growth is key to timing and sequencing of orthodontic intervention, third molar extractions, re-establishment of vertical dimension, or placement of an esthetic anterior implant. A knowledgeable dental professional may be able to assist their adolescent patients with eating disorders through regularly scheduled recall examinations.

CLINICS CARE POINTS

- Nutrition is the key component that contributes to steady growth and development during adolescence.
- Regardless of the eating disorder, the essential first phase of treatment is to initiate a meticulous home care regimen, which includes brushing and flossing.
- The second phase of treatment includes scheduling more frequent recall appointments so that the dentist can monitor patient compliance, provide additional professional services, and have the opportunity to discover hard- and soft-tissue changes at earlier stages to initiate more conservative treatment.
- An additional phase of treatment may be referral to dental specialists, pediatricians, primary care providers, mental health professionals, or nutrition specialists.

DISCLOSURE

The authors have nothing to disclose.

REFERENCES

1. Franzini Pereira R, Alvarenga M. Disordered eating: identifying, treating, preventing, and differentiating it from eating disorders. Diabetes Spectr 2007;30:141–8.
2. Watt RG. Correspondence: COVID-19 is an opportunity for reform in dentistry. Lancet 2020;396:462.
3. Golden NH, Katzman DK. Anorexia nervosa. In: Fisher MM, Alderman EM, Kreipe RE, et al, editors. Textbook of adolescent health care. Itasca, (IL): American Academy of Pediatrics; 2011. p. 743–58.
4. Smink FRE, van Hoeken D, Hoek HW. Epidemiology of eating disorders: Incidence, prevalence and mortality rates. Curr Psychiatry Rep 2012;14:406–14.
5. Cooper M, Reilly EE, Siegel JA, et al. Eating disorders during the COVID-19 pandemic: an overview of risks and recommendations for treatment and early intervention. Eat Disord 2020;1–23.
6. American Psychiatric Association. Feeding and eating disorders. In: Diagnostic and statistical manual of mental disorders (DSM–5). 5th edition. Arlington, VA: American Psychiatric Association; 2013. p. 338–54.
7. American Psychiatric Association. Feeding and eating disorders. In: Diagnostic and statistical manual of mental disorders (DSM–4) Text Revision. 4th edition. Arlington, VA: American Psychiatric Association; 2000. p. 583–95.
8. Berrettini W. The genetics of eating disorders. Psychiatry 2004;(3):18–25.
9. Hellstrom I. Anorexia nervosa-ontogenic problems. Swed Dent J 1974;67:253–69.

10. Holst J, Lang F. Perimlolysis? A contribution towards the genesis of tooth wasting from non-mechanical causes. Acta Odont Scand 1939;1:36–48.

11. Ranalli DN, Rye L. Oral health issues for women athletes. Dent Clin North Am 2001;45(3):523–39.

12. Jeffcoat MK, Chestnut CH. Systemic osteoporosis and oral bone loss: Evidence shows increased risk factors. J Am Dent Assoc 1993;124:49–56.

13. Otis CL, Drinkwater B, Johnson M, et al. The female athlete triad. American College of Sports Medicine position stand. Med Sci Sports Exerc 1997;29(5):i–ix.

14. Nazem TG, Ackerman KE. The female athlete triad. Sports Health 2012;4(4): 302–11.

15. Nattiv A, Loucks AB, Manore MM, et al. American College of Sports Medicine. The female athlete triad. Med Sci Sports Exerc 2007;39(10):1867–82.

16. Rome ES. The female athlete triad. In: Fisher MM, Alderman EM, Kreipe RE, et al, editors. Textbook of adolescent health care. Itasca, (IL): American Academy of Pediatrics; 2011. p. 770–7.

17. Hoch AZ, Pajewski NM, Moraski L, et al. Prevalence of the female athlete triad in high school athletes and sedentary students. Clin J Sport Med 2009;19(5):421–8.

18. Nichols JF, Rauh MJ, Lawson MJ, et al. Prevalence of the female athlete triad syndrome among high school athletes. Arch Pediatr Adolesc Med 2006;160(2): 137–42.

19. Barrack MT, Ackerman KE, Gibbs JC. Update on the female athlete triad. Curr Rev Musculoskelet Med 2013;6(2):195–204.

20. Fredericson M, Kent K. Normalization of bone density in a previously amenorrheic runner with osteoporosis. Med Sci Sports Exerc 2005;37(9):1481–6.

21. Gibbs JC, Williams NI, De Souza MJ. Prevalence of individual and combined components of the female athlete triad. Med Sci Sports Exerc 2013;45(5):985–96.

22. Hind K. Recovery of bone mineral density and fertility in a former amenorrheic athlete. J Sports Sci Med 2008;7(3):415–8.

23. Russell G. Bulimia nervosa: an ominous variant of anorexia nervosa. Psychol Med 1979;9:429–48.

24. Brown C, Mehler PS. Medical complications of self-induced vomiting. J Eat Disord 2013;21:287–94.

25. Mehler PS, Rylander M. Bulimia nervosa – medical complications. J Eat Disord 2015;3:12.

26. Winstead N, Willard S. Gastrointestinal complaints in patients with eating disorders. J Clin Gastroenterol 2006;40:678–82.

27. Little J. Eating disorders: dental implications. Oral Radiol Endod 2008;106: 696–707.

28. Mehler PS. Medical complications of bulimia nervosa and their treatments. Int J Eat Disord 2011;44:95–104.

29. Mignogna M, Fedele S, Russo L. Anorexia/bulimia – related sialadenosis of palatal minor salivary glands. J Oral Pathol Med 2004;33:441–2.

30. Centers for Disease Control and Prevention. Childhood obesity facts. Available at: https://www.cdc.gov/obesity/data/childhood.html. Accessed May 12, 2021.

31. Wisniewski AB, Chernausek SD. Gender in childhood obesity: family environment, hormones, and genes. Gend Med 2009;6(Suppl 1):76–85.

32. Rieder J, Salazar A. Obesity. In: Fisher MM, Alderman EM, Kreipe RE, et al, editors. Textbook of adolescent health care. American Academy of Pediatrics; 2011. p. 778–89.

33. Golden NH, Schneider M, Wood C. Committee on nutrition, committee on adolescence, and section on obesity. Pediatrics 2016;138(3):e20161649.

34. Tirosh A, Shai I, Afek A, et al. Adolescent BMI trajectory and risk of diabetes versus coronary disease. N Engl J Med 2011;364:1315–25.
35. Whitlock EP, Williams SB, Gold R, et al. Screening and interventions for childhood overweight: a summary of evidence for the US Preventive Services Task Force. Pediatrics 2005;116:e125–44.
36. Strauss RS, Pollack HA. Social marginalization of overweight children. Arch Pediatr Adolesc Med 2003;157:746–52.
37. National Eating Disorders. Binge eating disorder. Available at: https://www.nationaleatingdisorders.org/learn/by-eating-disorder/bed. Accessed May 12, 2021.
38. Paisi M, Kay E, Bennett C, et al. Body mass index and dental caries in young people: a systematic review. BMC Pediatr 2019;19:122.
39. Kang J, Vann WF Jr, Lee JY, et al. The safety of sedation for overweight/obese children in the dental setting. Pediatr Dent 2012;34:392–6.
40. Aissaoui A, Salem NH, Mougou M, et al. Dental age assessment among Tunisian children using the Demirjian method. J Forensic Dent Sci 2016;8:47–51.
41. Sopher AB, Jean AM, Zwany SK, et al. Bone age advancement in prepubertal children with obesity and premature adrenarche: possible potentiating factors. Obesity 2011;19:1259–64.
42. Brown JJ, Warne GL. Growth in precocious puberty. Indian J Pediatr 2006; 73:81–8.
43. Nicholas CL, Kadavy K, Holton NE, et al. Childhood body mass index is associated with early dental development and eruption in a longitudinal sample from the Iowa Facial Growth Study. Am J Orthod Dentofacial Orthop 2018;154:72–81.
44. Chehab DA, Tanbonliong T, Peyser J, et al. Association between body mass index and dental age in Hispanic children. Gen Den 2017;65:54–8.
45. Omar S, Oyoyo U, Alfi W, et al. Relationship between body mass index and dental development in a contemporary pediatric population in the United States. J Dent Child 2019;86:93–100.
46. Saito T, Shimazaki Y, Sakamoto M. Obesity and periodontitis. N Engl J Med 1998; 339:482–3.
47. Maciel SS, Feres M, Goncalves TED, et al. Does obesity influence the subgingival microbiota composition in periodontal health and disease? J Clin Periodontol 2016;43:1003–12.
48. Modeer T, Blomberg C, Wondimu B, et al. Association between obesity and periodontal risk indicators in adolescents. Intl J Pediatr Obes 2011;6:e264–70.
49. Ritchie C. Obesity and periodontal disease. Periodontol 2000 2007;44:154–63.
50. Saito T, Shimazaki Y, Koga T, et al. Relationship between upper body obesity and periodontitis. J Dent Res 2001;80:1631–6.
51. Al-Zahrani MS, Bissaa NG, Borawskit EA. Obesity and periodontal disease in young, middle-aged, and older adults. J Periodontol 2003;74:610–5.
52. Kershaw EE, Flier JS. Adipose tissue as an endocrine organ. J Clin Endocrinol Metab 2004;89:2548–56.
53. Pischon N, Heng N, Bernimoulin J-P, et al. Obesity, inflammation, and periodontal disease. J Dent Res 2007;86(5):400–9.
54. Marro F, De Smedt S, Rajasekharan S, et al. Associations between obesity, dental caries, erosive tooth wear and periodontal disease in adolescents: a case-control study. Eur Arch Paediatr Dent 2021;22:99–108.
55. de Andrade PAM, Giovani PA, Araujo DA, et al. Shifts in the bacterial community of saliva give insights on the relationship between obesity and oral microbiota in adolescents. Arch Microbiol 2020;202:1085–95.

Understanding and Caring for LGBTQ+ Youth by the Oral Health Care Provider

Joshua A. Raisin, DDS[a], Deanna Adkins, MD[b],
Scott B. Schwartz, DDS, MPH[c,d,*]

KEYWORDS

- LGBT • Transgender • Adolescents • Oral health • Disparities • Best practices

KEY POINTS

- An increasing prevalence of LGBTQ+ youth accentuates the need for oral health providers to have a deeper understanding of the etiology and implications of sexuality and gender development.
- LGBTQ+ youth face a number of health disparities that impact both oral and overall health.
- There are nuances to treating LGBTQ+ youth that can improve the oral health care experience for this vulnerable population.

INTRODUCTION

With increasing visibility, individuals who are lesbian, gay, bisexual, transgender, queer, intersex, two-spirited, or something else (LGBTQ+) are more empowered to publicly identify this way, particularly among younger generations. Current estimates from national surveys indicate that roughly 9% of United States (US) youth aged 13 to 17 years identify as lesbian, gay, or bisexual (LGB) and 0.73% identify as transgender.[1] Despite the trend to more freely express diverse sexual orientations and gender identities, LGBTQ+ individuals of all ages continue to experience misconceptions, discrimination, and widespread health disparities.

[a] Division of Pediatric and Public Health, University of North Carolina Adams School of Dentistry, 228 Brauer Hall, CB 7450, Chapel Hill, NC 27599-7450, USA; [b] Division of Endocrinology and Metabolism, Department of Pediatrics, Duke University School of Medicine, 3000 Erwin Road, DUMC 102820, Durham, NC 27710, USA; [c] Department of Pediatrics, University of Cincinnati – College of Medicine, Cincinnati, OH, USA; [d] Division of Pediatric Dentistry and Orthodontics, Cincinnati Children's Hospital Medical Center, 3333 Burnet Avenue, MLC 2006, Cincinnati, OH 45229, USA
* Corresponding author. 3333 Burnet Avenue, MLC 2006, Cincinnati, OH 45229.
E-mail address: scott.schwartz@cchmc.org

Dent Clin N Am 65 (2021) 705–717
https://doi.org/10.1016/j.cden.2021.06.007
0011-8532/21/© 2021 Elsevier Inc. All rights reserved.

Dental and allied oral health educational programs provide inadequate training on these topics, generally relegating the discussion to review pathologies that may be prevalent in this population without presentation of other pertinent characteristics. However, a deeper understanding of LGBTQ+ youth can improve the overall health care experience for these patients, their families, and their providers. Therefore, this review intends to provide background information on sexuality and gender development, an overview of transgender medicine, LGBTQ+ health disparities, and the implications for oral health care.

DEVELOPMENT OF SEXUAL ORIENTATION AND GENDER IDENTITY
Development of Sexual Orientation

Sexual orientation refers to one's pattern of romantic, emotional, and physical attractions and their relation to the gender(s) of the person to whom they are attracted to (**Fig. 1**). Sexual identity development, similar to gender identity development, is discovered over time. There are multiple dimensions to one's sexuality that minimally include attraction, interest, orientation, and behaviors. The sexual and romantic aspects of this may also be different from each other within the same individual. Awareness of attraction is often first observed or tends to occur in early adolescence, which is around age 9 for those assigned female at birth and around 10 for those assigned male at birth. Youth who identify as anything other than heterosexual may experience this attraction later.[2] This phase of young adulthood includes becoming aware of these parts of their identity via attraction, fantasies, and behavior.[3] In addition, this age group has more concrete thinking, discomfort with their developing body changes from puberty, and interest in exploring some sexual behaviors.

Adolescents' uncertainty about their sexual orientation decreases with age, from 26% of 12-year-old students to 5% of 17-year-olds.[4] Approximately 5% to 10% of teens identify as LGB. However, over 10% of females and between 2% and 6% of males report having participated in same-gender sexual activity.[5]

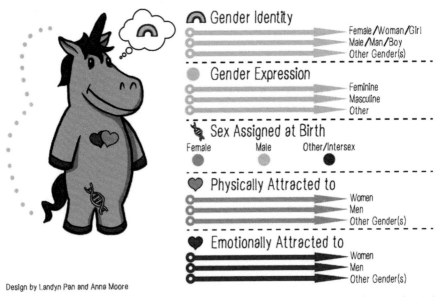

Design by Landyn Pan and Anna Moore

Fig. 1. The Gender Unicorn. (*From* Trans Student Educational Resources. "The Gender Unicorn." 2015. www.transstudent.org/gender. Accessed April 25, 2021.)

Development of Gender Identity

Gender identity is one's inner sense of their gender, which may or may not match the sex assigned at birth. Sex assigned at birth is a designation primarily made on visual inspection of external genitalia. When these 2 align, one is cisgender. When they do not align, one is transgender. Gender identity is often thought to exist on a spectrum between the binary poles of male and female, but more likely, gender identity exists in more of a cloud. There are many ways that a person can identify with regard to their gender.

- Most common gender identities are male and female.
- Other common gender identities are nonbinary, genderqueer, and agender.
- Additional gender identities exist and are personal to each individual.

Gender identity is a normal part of childhood development and occurs through several time points.

Birth to age five

In the earliest stage, children commonly explore their gender by looking at their bodies and comparing them to other children. They also observe how adults act with one another and how they treat children based on gender. During this time, children will often try out different gender expressions by dressing up in clothes that may not match their gender assignment. Parents may be concerned or confused when this occurs; however, this is normal and does not necessarily correlate with their adult gender identity. This behavior should simply be treated as play. A small minority of transgender children present at this age. These children are very consistent, persistent, and insistent that their gender was assigned incorrectly. The longer this insistence continues, the more likely that the child will continue to identify as transgender as an adult.[6]

Age five to onset of puberty

From age 5 until the onset of puberty, gender exploration is typically more quiescent. Generally, puberty begins around age 9 in those assigned female at birth and 11 and a half in those assigned male at birth. Pubertal onset and sex hormone production serves as a trigger for robust gender and sexual identity development. Sometimes, these 2 distinct identities may be confused, and one such adolescent may require time to sort them out. At this stage, a small subset of youth may develop gender dysphoria, defined as a significant discomfort with the lack of alignment between their assigned gender and their gender identity. Should more time for exploration be necessary, it is possible to pause puberty using gonadotropin-releasing hormone (GnRH) antagonists to allow further understanding of their true identity.[7,8] The GnRH antagonists leuprolide and histrelin help by temporarily halting development of secondary sexual characteristics, such as breast development or body hair growth, among others. Placing a pause on puberty can facilitate avoiding surgery such as a mastectomy as an adult. Additional benefits include relieving gender dysphoria, improving quality of life, and reducing anxiety, depression, self-harm, and suicidal ideation.[9] There can be a transient decrease in bone density while on GnRH antagonists, but this normalizes or stabilizes after the addition of gender-affirming hormones or discontinuing the GnRH antagonist.[10]

Puberty

Puberty can be unpaused without any long-term consequences. If the youth no longer identifies as transgender, simply removing the suppressant will allow their endogenous pubertal axis to proceed as normal. However, if they persist in their identification as transgender, then they can continue on to gender-affirming hormones at the appropriate time for a typical "late bloomer."

After puberty

Most transgender youth present in late puberty or late adolescence. Still others may not come out until they are much older. In this case, these individuals would bypass GnRH antagonists and initiate gender-affirming hormones should they choose to hormonally transition. Consolidation of gender identity occurs in late adolescence. There may be some changes that are minor after that time with regard to expression or nuances in identity, but it is highly unlikely for someone to identify as cisgender if they have identified as transgender at this stage of development.

Sexual orientation, sex assigned at birth, and gender identity are often confused. The Gender Unicorn (**Fig. 1**), helps to illustrate their definition and how these are related to each other.

Transgender Youth and Transitioning: Stages and Types of Transition

Although understanding of one's identity continues throughout life, a person's understanding of their gender identity is generally stable after adolescence. This does not mean that people only truly are transgender if they transition or come out in adolescence as there are many reasons that person may not transition until later in life. Transitioning and gender affirmation allows transgender individuals to live life according to their internal sense of gender and ultimately decreases anxiety and depression.[11] There are 3 distinct phases of the transition process, and individuals may elect to participate in all, some, or none of these phases.

Social transition

The first, and completely reversible, phase of transition is often a social transition. It can include a number of changes that are culturally specific regarding typical gender expression. In the United States, for example, it is common for boys to have short hair, wear plain pants and shirts, and avoid nail polish and makeup. Girls, on the other hand, frequently have long hair, wear bright or ornamental clothing, and are interested in cosmetics. Thus, an individual assigned male at birth identifying as a girl may grow their hair out and opt for dresses at school. These decisions about outward presentation may change over time. In addition to changes in appearance, the social transition may include selection of a different name and pronouns.

Sometimes social transitioning occurs before the medical transition, other times it occurs concurrently. What matters for most youth is that the provider asks about their personal perspective, experience, and what terminology best suits their needs.

Medical transition

Medical transition is when a person uses gender-affirming hormones that match their gender identity to better match that identity physically. This is a very effective method of improving alignment between body and identity and leads to relief of dysphoria and related depression and anxiety. Overall improvement in quality of life, depression, and anxiety is nearly 80% with this process.[12]

It is important to keep in mind the patient is on these medications and how they may or may not interact with any medications or procedures in your office. In general, the goal is to keep the hormone levels in the normal physiologic range for the gender they identify with and thus should not cause much interference. If there are questions or concerns, the dental team should feel empowered to engage with medical providers to ensure the best treatment for the transgender child, similar to any other patient with a health condition that may be affected by their dental procedures. Some of the relevant reported potential side effects of these medications are described in **Table 1**. No long-term adverse dental or oral outcomes are currently reported in the literature secondary to gender-affirming hormone use.

Surgical transition

Surgical transition is another method that a person who is transgender can use to better align their bodies with their gender identity. There are several procedures that can be done:

- For transgender women:
  a. Facial feminization
  b. Tracheal shave
  c. Vocal fold procedures
  d. Vaginoplasty
  e. Penectomy
  f. Orchiectomy
  g. Breast augmentation
- For transgender men:
  a. Mastectomy
  b. Metoidoplasty
  c. Phalloplasty
  d. Hysterectomy with or without complete oophorectomy
  e. Vaginectomy

These are very rarely performed in individuals younger than 18 years in the United States, although the age of consent varies elsewhere. Not all transgender individuals have a surgical transition because not everyone needs these procedures to feel comfortable with their bodies. Furthermore, they are expensive and often not covered by insurance. Some of these procedures are rather complex with a higher rate of complications than others which may serve as a reason one may not elect to have them. Additionally, local surgeons may not have expertize in these procedures which contributes to a long waitlist for those who do.

Other than understanding how a person tolerated anesthesia or if you are doing a procedure where a urinary catheter might need to be placed, it is unlikely that knowing

Table 1	
Potential side effects from medications used during transition	
Medications	**Side effects**
Estrogens	<ul><li>Increased risk for blood clots, specifically venous thromboembolism</li><li>Body fat redistribution</li><li>Decreased bone density and osteoporosis risk</li><li>Liver function changes</li></ul>
Androgen blockers (eg, spironolactone)	<ul><li>Dehydration</li><li>Elevated potassium, if severe, can lead to cardiac arrhythmias</li></ul>
Androgens (eg, testosterone)	<ul><li>Elevated hemoglobin</li><li>Liver function changes</li></ul>

Data from: Hembree, WC, Cohen-Kettenis, PT, Gooren, L, et al; Endocrine Treatment of Gender-Dysphoric/Gender-Incongruent Persons: An Endocrine Society Clinical Practice Guideline; J Clin Endocrinol Metab; 2017 Nov 1;102(11):3869-3903.

whether a patient has had one of these procedures would be pertinent to delivering dental care. Asking too many questions about a person's transition surgeries when they are not relevant is unnecessary and should be avoided.

LGBTQ+ Youth Health Disparities

Health disparities within the LGBTQ+ community are well-documented in literature. Research has demonstrated many possible reasons for these disparities: financial barriers to health care, difficulty finding affirmative providers, lack of social network and support, as well as lifetime victimization.[13–15] The Minority Stress Model is the leading explanatory theory for sexual orientation–related health disparities and suggests that members of a minority population experience persistent stress related to their sexual orientation.[16]

Minority stress may lead to poorer health through anticipated discrimination, actual experiences with prejudicial events, and internalized stigma. Anticipated discrimination refers to the expectation of being marginalized as a consequence of social stigma or past negative encounters in health care settings. Actual discrimination refers to the lived experience of LGBTQ+ individuals and can include situations such as health care providers making homophobic or transphobic comments or failing to recognize same-sex partners as family members.[17,18] Transgender people often delay seeking care and express distress with disclosing their gender identity to their provider.[19] Avoidance of health care, in part, may be attributed to internalized stigma. The way in which LGBTQ+ people experience discrimination may result in accepting the negative attitude toward them and choosing to avoid care.[17]

Ignorance around LGBTQ+-related health is another barrier preventing people from accessing care. Many LGBTQ+ people report being unable to discuss health issues that relate to their sexual orientation as a result of obvious displays of discomfort by their care providers.[18] According to the 2015 US Transgender Survey, 24% of respondents reported having to teach their provider about transgender people to receive appropriate care.[20] Several studies have illustrated the frustration and concerns transgender patients have with mental health professionals and their determination of eligibility for gender-confirming surgery.[21–23] There are insufficient data to support that health care professionals are adequately trained to provide appropriate care to the trans and nonbinary community.[24]

With the increasing prevalence of individuals identifying as trans and nonbinary, barriers to seeking transgender-related health care are slowly improving. Government health care programs (eg, Medicaid, Medicare) and private insurance plans have started to incorporate coverage for gender-affirming care and surgery.[25] However, many transgender and nonbinary individuals avoid seeking health care because of poor experiences. These have included insensitivity to one's gender identity, awkward interactions believed to be related to gender identity, refusal of care, substandard care, verbal abuse, and being forced to seek psychiatric treatment.[26]

Despite analyzing LGBTQ+ health disparities through federally funded health surveys, most do not gather information on gender identity.[27] Thus, obtaining information regarding transgender health is difficult, particularly as it pertains to transgender youth. It is understood, however, that transgender and nonbinary individuals have a higher odds of reporting poor physical and mental health relative to their cisgender counterparts.[28] They are often victim to various forms of stigma, discrimination, and exclusion in public settings and, as a consequence, experience high levels of psychological distress.[29] A history of antitransgender violence, or fear of it, may prevent an individual from seeking medical care.

The discrimination faced by LGBTQ+ youth may lead to an array of negative physical and mental health disorders. LGBTQ+ people often report being victim to verbal harassment and feeling unwelcome because of their sexual orientation and/or gender identity. Depression and suicidal ideation or attempts are common sequelae of such marginalization. LGBTQ+ youth are more likely than their cisgender and heterosexual counterparts to die by suicide related to the homophobia, biphobia, and transphobia they may experience in society.[30] Exclusion from society often includes parental rejection too. Approximately 30% to 45% of LGBTQ+ youth experience homelessness, which has also been associated with higher rates of mental health disorders and suicidality.[31–33] Homelessness makes obtaining care of any type, particularly preventive, difficult because of both cost and access.

Already faced with an array of mental health issues, the COVID-19 pandemic placed LGBTQ+ youth in a difficult situation, with some reporting difficulty being isolated with an unsupportive or unsafe family, removed from critical social connections, and less access to support staff and necessary medical care.[34,35] Online versions of real-time chat or voice counseling sessions have proven helpful for those who had access during quarantine.[34,35]

LGBTQ+ adolescents are more likely to engage in risky conduct, including substance use and abuse, tobacco smoking, and high-risk sexual behaviors.[19,36] They report a greater number of drinking days and heavy drinking episodes than their heterosexual, cisgender counterparts.[37] Tobacco use for LGB people is approximately twice as high compared with heterosexuals.[38] There are several risk-enhancing variables attached to this: being single, reporting more poor mental health days, excessive drinking, life dissatisfaction, low income, barriers to health care, unemployment, and so forth.[38] These behaviors are more associated with less-affirmative communities and schools.[37]

LGBTQ+ youth, especially men who have sex with men, show a high incidence of sexually transmitted diseases that can be attributed to earlier onset in sexual experiences, increased number of sexual encounters with multiple partners, and poor education on safe sex practices. According to the Center for Disease Control and Prevention data from 2018, gay and bisexual men comprised 69% of new HIV diagnoses for those aged 13 years and older.[39] The 2015 US Transgender Survey found the prevalence of HIV infection to be 5 times greater for trans and nonbinary individuals relative to the general population.[20]

Minimal research is available on oral health–specific disparities related to the LGBTQ+ community. One study noted an increased prevalence in oral human papilloma virus-positive status among gay and lesbian individuals relative to bisexual and heterosexual individuals. Moreover, LGB individuals reported higher prevalence of fair or poor oral health.[40] Another study showed transgender adults to be less likely to have visited the dentist in the past year compared to cisgender adults.[41] Trans and nonbinary people exhibit higher levels of dental fear as well.[42] Fortunately, transgender adolescents and young adults aged 14 years through 24 years have reported positive experiences with their oral health providers.[43] More oral health research is needed to properly assess the oral health status of LGBTQ+ youth.

Considerations for LGBTQ+ Youth in the Dental Setting

Dentists and allied providers receive limited training on LGBTQ+ health-related needs during formal training. One survey found 29% of participating US and Canadian dental schools reporting not covering LGBTQ+-related topics.[44] Another study revealed that only 13.3% of dental students felt adequately equipped to treat LGBTQ+ patients, which may be the result of minimal exposure in their clinical training.[45,46] Dental professionals who feel prepared, by their formal education, to treat people of diverse backgrounds are more likely to treat these patients in their communities.[47] Often, what is taught in dental curricula on LGBTQ+ people surround themes such as sexually transmitted diseases or substance use and abuse.[44] This information may be presented in a way that not only lacks discussion on how to address disparities with cultural competence but also further stigmatizes these populations. Fortunately, there are several evidence-based best practices when working with LGBTQ+ patients.

One challenge faced by caregivers of LGBTQ+ youth is finding accepting providers. Some may rely on social media or word-of-mouth to ascertain welcoming practices, while others are looking for indications on websites, promotional materials, or within the office.[43] Items such as a Safe Space sticker, pride flags or decals, and inclusive photos or magazines can all be ways to indicate the practice is welcoming to LGBTQ+ youth. Caregivers of transgender youth report carefully reviewing office nondiscrimination policies for protected terms such as "sexual orientation" and "gender identity." Inclusive language for intake forms and while conversing are important drivers of a positive health care experience.[43,48]

Intake and medical history forms with considerate and inclusive language can be the first sign of a welcoming practice. This includes detailed inquiries on gender identity, name, and pronoun preferences. A two-step method for identifying noncisgender individuals has been proposed, recording both the sex assigned at birth and the gender identity.[49] This way of collecting information has proven to be effective, as it takes into account the biological (ie, gender assigned at birth) and social (ie, gender identity) constructs.

It is vital for practitioners to be familiar with gender identities that extend beyond the traditional binary view. LGBTQ+ youth may have preferred pronouns correlating with their gender identity and not sex assigned at birth, thus making it important to also ask patients when obtaining a medical history.[50,51] Patients report greater satisfaction and less anxiety when they are addressed by their preferred name and pronouns.[43] Dentists are strongly encouraged to revise their intake forms to better reflect the needs of all genders and sexualities. An example of an inclusive intake form can be seen in **Fig. 2**.

The dentist and supporting staff should foster an environment welcoming youth and adolescents to speak freely of their sexual and gender identities. Dentists should feel comfortable bringing up visible changes and discussing gender identity, as the patient may be unsure of how to initiate this conversation.[52] However, transgender youth express little reason to disclose their transition-related health matters, such as medications, hormone therapies, and surgical procedures because they do not feel it is relevant to their oral health needs.[53]

It is especially important for dentists and personnel to be cognizant of the fact that a patient may be discovering their gender identity long before going through with affirmative care and, as such, should take extra caution with not assuming one's gender. Gender-neutral terminology helps to provide youth with an atraumatic dental visit. Dentists are also encouraged to periodically update gender status, preferred names, and pronouns, to allow for patients to disclose any updates.

Doctor-patient confidentiality is of utmost importance when these patients disclose their sexual and/or gender identities. Some adolescents may not disclose this type of information when still discovering their identity and when they lack parental support.[52] Dental professionals and personnel should understand that it is not their responsibility to inform caregivers of this information unless they are placing themselves in danger. However, the dental team is encouraged to be supportive of caregiver's feelings and should aid in finding resources to help them adjust and accept their child's identity.[51]

Child's Name (as it appears on birth certificate or insurance card): _____

Child's Preferred Name: _____ Preferred Pronouns?_____ Birth Date_____ Age____

Who is/are the legal guardian(s) of the child?:_____ and _____

Who is completing this form?:_____ Relation to Child?_____

Parent/Guardian Contact information: Home Phone (   )_____ Work (   ) _____ Cell (   ) _____

Email address:_____ __   Addn'l Phone (   )_____   (   )_____

Primary Care(Pediatrician)/Family Doctor Name/Practice:_____ Phone:_____

Referring Provider to this clinic: _____ Phone:_____

What is your Child's Gender Identity:
(Please check as many as apply)

☐ Male
☐ Female
☐ Transgender Male (FTM)
☐ Transgender Female (MTF)
☐ Gender queer or Gender fluid
☐ Agender
☐ Questioning
☐ Decline to Answer

Child's sex assigned at birth (check one) :

☐ Male   ☐ Intersex
☐ Female   ☐ Decline to Answer

Child's Race/Ethnicity:
(Please check as many as apply)

☐ American Indian or Alaskan   ☐ Hispanic
☐ Black, not of Hispanic origin   ☐ Asian
☐ White, not of Hispanic origin   ☐ Pacific Islander
☐ Decline to Answer   ☐ Native Hawaiian

Fig. 2. Sample intake form. (*Courtesy of* Duke Child and Adolescent Gender Care Clinic; with permission.)

Should a dentist feel unequipped to meet a patient's needs themselves, they should be aware of LGBTQ+-affirming providers in the community.[48]

SUMMARY

It is especially important to have LGBTQ+-affirming dentists and staff in the community that are well educated on all aspects of LGBTQ+-related needs, including an understanding of sexual behaviors, oral health susceptibilities, and gender-affirming care. Minor changes to the clinic routine and a deeper understanding of this unique population can improve both care for the patient and facilitate a more profound patient-provider relationship.

DISCLOSURE STATEMENT

The authors have nothing to disclose.

CLINICS CARE POINTS

- Parents of LGBTQ+ youth are frequently looking for signs of an experienced and accepting dentist.
- Modifications to intake forms, LGBTQ+-related flags or images, and awareness of gendered language can make LGBTQ+ youth feel more comfortable in the dental setting.

- Elevated prevalence of risky health behaviors among LGBTQ+ youth, such as substance use and abuse and early sexual contact, can directly impact oral health.

REFERENCES

1. Conron KJ. LGBT Youth Population in the United States. The Williams Institute, UCLA. Available at: https://williamsinstitute.law.ucla.edu/publications/lgbt-youth-pop-us/. Accessed April 25, 2020.
2. Herdt GH, Boxer A. Children of horizons: how gay and lesbian teens are leading a new way out of the closet. Boston: Beacon Press; 1996.
3. Mustanski B, Birkett M, Greene GJ, et al. The association between sexual orientation identity and behavior across race/ethnicity, sex, and age in a probability sample of high school students. Am J Public Health 2014; 104(2):237–44.
4. Remafedi G, Resnick M, Blum R, et al. Demography of sexual orientation in adolescents. Pediatrics 1992;89(4):714–21.
5. Kann L, Olsen EO, McManus T, et al. Sexual identity, sex of sexual contacts, and health-risk behaviors among students in grades 9-12–youth risk behavior surveillance, selected sites, United States, 2001-2009. MMWR Surveill Summ 2011; 60(7):1–133.
6. Leibowitz SF, Telingator C. Assessing gender identity concerns in children and adolescents: evaluation, treatments, and outcomes. Curr Psychiatry Rep 2012; 14(2):111–20.
7. de Vries AL, Steensma TD, Doreleijers TA, et al. Puberty suppression in adolescents with gender identity disorder: a prospective follow-up study. J Sex Med 2011;8(8):2276–83.
8. Kreukels BP, Cohen-Kettenis PT. Puberty suppression in gender identity disorder: the Amsterdam experience. Nat Rev Endocrinol 2011;7(8):466–72.
9. Turban JL, King D, Carswell JM, et al. Pubertal Suppression for Transgender Youth and Risk of Suicidal Ideation. Pediatrics 2020;145(2). https://doi.org/10. 1542/peds.2019-1725.
10. Vlot MC, Klink DT, den Heijer M, et al. Effect of pubertal suppression and cross-sex hormone therapy on bone turnover markers and bone mineral apparent density (BMAD) in transgender adolescents. Bone 2017;95:11–9.
11. Fontanari AMV, Vilanova F, Schneider MA, et al. Gender Affirmation Is Associated with Transgender and Gender Nonbinary Youth Mental Health Improvement. LGBT Health 2020;7(5):237–47.
12. Hembree WC, Cohen-Kettenis PT, Gooren L, et al. Endocrine Treatment of Gender-Dysphoric/Gender-Incongruent Persons: An Endocrine Society Clinical Practice Guideline. J Clin Endocrinol Metab 2017;102(11):3869–903.
13. Dahlhamer JM, Galinsky AM, Joestl SS, et al. Barriers to Health Care Among Adults Identifying as Sexual Minorities: A US National Study. Am J Public Health 2016;106(6):1116–22.
14. Fredriksen-Goldsen KI, Emlet CA, Kim HJ, et al. The physical and mental health of lesbian, gay male, and bisexual (LGB) older adults: the role of key health indicators and risk and protective factors. Gerontologist 2013;53(4):664–75.
15. Gahagan J, Subirana-Malaret M. Improving pathways to primary health care among LGBTQ populations and health care providers: key findings from Nova Scotia, Canada. Int J Equity Health 2018;17(1):76.

16. Meyer IH. Prejudice, social stress, and mental health in lesbian, gay, and bisexual populations: conceptual issues and research evidence. Psychol Bull 2003; 129(5):674.

17. Casey LS, Reisner SL, Findling MG, et al. Discrimination in the United States: Experiences of lesbian, gay, bisexual, transgender, and queer Americans. Health Serv Res 2019;54(Suppl 2):1454–66.

18. Lee A, Kanji Z. Queering the health care system: Experiences of the lesbian, gay, bisexual, transgender community. Can J Dental Hyg 2017;51(2):80–9.

19. Macapagal K, Bhatia R, Greene GJ. Differences in Healthcare Access, Use, and Experiences Within a Community Sample of Racially Diverse Lesbian, Gay, Bisexual, Transgender, and Questioning Emerging Adults. LGBT Health 2016; 3(6):434–42.

20. James S, Herman J, Rankin S, et al. The Report of the 2015 U.S. Transgender Survey. Washington, DC: National Center for Transgender Equality. Available at: https://transequality.org/sites/default/files/docs/usts/USTS-Full-Report-Dec17.pdf.

21. Bockting W, Robinson B, Benner A, et al. Patient satisfaction with transgender health services. J Sex Marital Ther 2004;30(4):277–94.

22. Wylie KR, Fitter J, Bragg A. The experience of service users with regard to satisfaction with clinical services. Sex Relationship Ther 2009;24(2):163–74.

23. Erasmus J, Bagga H, Harte F. Assessing patient satisfaction with a multidisciplinary gender dysphoria clinic in Melbourne. Australas Psychiatry 2015;23(2): 158–62.

24. Smith JR, Washington AZ 3rd, Morrison SD, et al. Assessing Patient Satisfaction Among Transgender Individuals Seeking Medical Services. Ann Plast Surg 2018; 81(6):725–9.

25. Zaliznyak M, Jung EE, Bresee C, et al. Which U.S. States' Medicaid Programs Provide Coverage for Gender-Affirming Hormone Therapy and Gender-Affirming Genital Surgery for Transgender Patients?: A State-by-State Review, and a Study Detailing the Patient Experience to Confirm Coverage of Services. J Sex Med 2021;18(2):410–22.

26. Kosenko K, Rintamaki L, Raney S, et al. Transgender patient perceptions of stigma in health care contexts. Med Care 2013;51(9):819–22.

27. Stroumsa D. The state of transgender health care: policy, law, and medical frameworks. Am J Public Health 2014;104(3):e31–8.

28. Lagos D. Looking at Population Health Beyond "Male" and "Female": Implications of Transgender Identity and Gender Nonconformity for Population Health. Demography 2018;55(6):2097–117.

29. Reisner SL, Hughto JM, Dunham EE, et al. Legal Protections in Public Accommodations Settings: A Critical Public Health Issue for Transgender and Gender-Nonconforming People. Milbank Q 2015;93(3):484–515.

30. Ream GL. What's unique about lesbian, gay, bisexual, and transgender (LGBT) youth and young adult suicides? Findings from the National Violent Death Reporting System. J Adolesc Health 2019;64(5):602–7.

31. Corliss HL, Goodenow CS, Nichols L, et al. High burden of homelessness among sexual-minority adolescents: findings from a representative Massachusetts high school sample. Am J Public Health 2011;101(9):1683–9.

32. Rhoades H, Rusow JA, Bond D, et al. Homelessness, Mental Health and Suicidality Among LGBTQ Youth Accessing Crisis Services. Child Psychiatry Hum Dev 2018;49(4):643–51.

33. Rice E, Fulginiti A, Winetrobe H, et al. Sexuality and homelessness in Los Angeles public schools. Am J Public Health 2012;102(2):200–1 [author reply: 202].

34. Fish JN, McInroy LB, Paceley MS, et al. "I'm Kinda Stuck at Home With Unsupportive Parents Right Now": LGBTQ Youths' Experiences With COVID-19 and the Importance of Online Support. J Adolesc Health 2020;67(3):450–2.

35. Salerno JP, Devadas J, Pease M, et al. Sexual and Gender Minority Stress Amid the COVID-19 Pandemic: Implications for LGBTQ Young Persons' Mental Health and Well-Being. Public Health Rep 2020;135(6):721–7.

36. Hafeez H, Zeshan M, Tahir MA, et al. Health Care Disparities Among Lesbian, Gay, Bisexual, and Transgender Youth: A Literature Review. Cureus 2017;9(4): e1184.

37. Coulter RW, Birkett M, Corliss HL, et al. Associations between LGBTQ-affirmative school climate and adolescent drinking behaviors. Drug Alcohol Depend 2016; 161:340–7.

38. Balsam KF, Beadnell B, Riggs KR. Understanding sexual orientation health disparities in smoking: a population-based analysis. Am J Orthop 2012;82(4): 482–93.

39. Centers for Disease Control and Prevention. HIV Surveillance Report, 2018 (Updated); vol. 31. Available at: https://stacks.cdc.gov/view/cdc/87803. Accessed April 25, 2021.

40. Schwartz SB, Sanders AE, Lee JY, et al. Sexual orientation-related oral health disparities in the United States. J Public Health Dent 2019;79(1):18–24. https://doi.org/10.1111/jphd.12290.

41. Hatzenbuehler ML, Birkett M, Van Wagenen A, et al. Protective school climates and reduced risk for suicide ideation in sexual minority youths. Am J Public Health 2014;104(2):279–86.

42. Heima M, Heaton LJ, Ng HH, et al. Dental fear among transgender individuals - a cross-sectional survey. Spec Care Dentist 2017;37(5):212–22.

43. Macdonald DW, Grossoehme DH, Mazzola A, et al. "I just want to be treated like a normal person": Oral health care experiences of transgender adolescents and young adults. J Am Dent Assoc 2019;150(9):748–54.

44. Hillenburg KL, Murdoch-Kinch CA, Kinney JS, et al. LGBT Coverage in U.S. Dental Schools and Dental Hygiene Programs: Results of a National Survey. J Dent Educ 2016;80(12):1440–9.

45. Anderson JI, Patterson AN, Temple HJ, et al. Lesbian, gay, bisexual, and transgender (LGBT) issues in dental school environments: dental student leaders' perceptions. J Dent Educ 2009;73(1):105–18.

46. Nowaskie DZ, Patel AU, Fang RC. A multicenter, multidisciplinary evaluation of 1701 healthcare professional students' LGBT cultural competency: Comparisons between dental, medical, occupational therapy, pharmacy, physical therapy, physician assistant, and social work students. PLoS One 2020;15(8):e0237670.

47. Smith CS, Ester TV, Inglehart MR. Dental education and care for underserved patients: an analysis of students' intentions and alumni behavior. J Dent Educ 2006; 70(4):398–408.

48. Romanelli M, Hudson KD. Individual and systemic barriers to health care: Perspectives of lesbian, gay, bisexual, and transgender adults. Am J Orthop 2017; 87(6):714–28.

49. Deutsch MB, Buchholz D. Electronic health records and transgender patients–practical recommendations for the collection of gender identity data. J Gen Intern Med 2015;30(6):843–7.

50. Aisner AJ, Zappas M, Marks A. Primary Care for Lesbian, Gay, Bisexual, Transgender, and Queer/Questioning (LGBTQ) Patients. J Nurse Pract 2020;16(4): 281–5.

51. Levine DA. Office-based care for lesbian, gay, bisexual, transgender, and questioning youth. Pediatrics 2013;132(1):e297–313.
52. Sequeira GM, Ray KN, Miller E, et al. Transgender Youth's Disclosure of Gender Identity to Providers Outside of Specialized Gender Centers. J Adolesc Health 2020;66(6):691–8.
53. Macdonald DW, Grossoehme DH, Mazzola A, et al. Transgender youth and oral health: a qualitative study. J LGBT Youth 2020;1–15.

Transitioning Adolescent Patients with Special Health Care Needs from Pediatric to Adult Dental Care

Karin Weber-Gasparoni, DDS, MS, PhD

KEYWORDS

- Adolescents • Children with special health care needs • Dental
- Health care transition

KEY POINTS

- Adequate dental training is needed to increase the number of qualified dentists that can treat individuals with special health care needs (SHCNs) when they age out from pediatrics.
- There is a paucity in the dental literature regarding transition policies and protocols from pediatric-centered to adult-centered care for individuals with SHCNs.
- There are significant disparities in race/ethnicity, socioeconomic status, and health status among individuals with SHCNs who do not achieve successful health care transition.
- Research is needed to evaluate transition protocols/strategies and assess their impact on oral health outcomes among individuals with SHCNs.

INTRODUCTION

The topic of transitioning patients from a pediatric to an adult health care team has gained worldwide visibility in both medical and dental fields over the past 2 decades.[1–18] Health care transition (HCT) from adolescence into adulthood is a complex and often disorganized process that lacks care coordination, care planning, collaboration, and communication between the pediatric and adult health care teams.[5] Adolescents and young adults are among the many vulnerable populations at risk for unhealthy behaviors, such as low medical and dental care utilization, poor dietary and oral hygiene, as well as smoking and drug use.[11,14]

Within this young population, individuals with special health care needs (SHCNs) are the most vulnerable.[9,19] The transition to adult health care is significantly more challenging and difficult to manage for young adults with SHCNs than for their healthier

Department of Pediatric Dentistry, University of Iowa, 202 Dental Science South, Iowa City, IA 52242-1001, USA
E-mail address: karin-weber@uiowa.edu

Dent Clin N Am 65 (2021) 719–729
https://doi.org/10.1016/j.cden.2021.06.010
dental.theclinics.com

peers.[5–17] After aging out of the pediatric health care system, a large number of these patients "drop out" of the health care system, with no responsible primary care provider to guide them into adulthood.[2] Regardless of their age, individuals with SHCNs have more unmet health and dental needs, along with more barriers to accessing adequate medical and dental care.[9,20] In fact, dental care is considered the most common unmet health care need among individuals with SHCNs.[21]

A definition of SHCN states that "special health care needs include any physical, developmental, mental, sensory, behavioral, cognitive, or emotional impairment or limiting condition that requires medical management, health care intervention, and/or use of specialized services or programs. The condition may be congenital, developmental, or acquired through disease, trauma, or environmental cause and may impose limitations in performing daily self-maintenance activities or substantial limitations in a major life activity. Health care for individuals with special needs requires specialized knowledge, as well as increased awareness and attention, adaptation, and accommodative measures beyond what are considered routine."[22]

A national report has shown that in 2019, 13.2% of the total civilian population in the United States (US) had one or more reported disabilities,[23] with the prevalence of disabilities increasing with age.[24] In 2019, over 3 million children had a disability in the US, which represented 4.3% of the population under the age of 18 years.[25] Higher rates of disability were observed with an increase in age: less than 1% of children under the age of 5 years, 5.5% of children aged 5 to 14 years, and 6.1% of children aged 15 to 17 years.[25] Advances in science and pediatric health care have dramatically improved the survival rate of patients with SHCNs. It is estimated that 90% of individuals with SHCNs and chronic conditions who require specialized medical and dental care live into adulthood.[26] Consequently, there is a need to successfully transition these patients into the adult health care system to receive comprehensive care that is medically and developmentally appropriate for their age and complex needs. It has been reported that individuals with SHCNs who have successfully transitioned are more likely to receive continuous care, which has the greatest positive impact on their long-term health outcomes.[8]

HEALTH CARE TRANSITION
Definition and Goals

HCT is defined as "the purposeful, planned movement of adolescents and young adults with chronic physical and medical conditions from child-centered to adult-oriented health care systems."[1] The goals of HCT for young adults with and without SHCNs are to optimize their health and lifelong functioning by providing uninterrupted and high-quality health care.[6] All adolescents and young adults should have a timely and individualized HCT plan, regardless of their health care needs status. For HCT to be effective, it should be regarded as a dynamic planning process involving a collaborative team (ie, patient, caregivers, physicians, dentists, social workers) and a series of organized steps, rather than a one-time isolated event.[6] The planning and support for HCT should be initiated early and be part of the routine primary care for all adolescents.[14] The initial discussion about HCT between a youth and their caregivers should be initiated when the child is 12 years of age, with the ultimate goal of finalizing the transition by 18 to 21 years of age.[6,7]

For individuals with SHCNs, developing an HCT might require a more extended transition plan than for those without SHCNs. An HCT for individuals with SHCNs may include, but is not limited to, an exchange of information between the pediatric and adult health care team about the patient's complex medical needs, need for comanagement, special accommodations, intellectual and self-care competencies, referrals to subspecialties, as well as issues on guardianship, informed consent, changes in the medical and dental insurance, and ineligibility for services previously covered during childhood.[7] Although HCT encourages young adults to take control of their own health and function as independently as possible, these expectations might not be fulfilled for patients with SHCNs, particularly for those whose cognitive and/or intellectual disabilities impair their ability for self-management and health promotion.

Guiding Principles

In order to achieve a successful HCT, it is important to consider the fundamental principles of transition that have been studied and are endorsed by national medical and dental organizations.[13–15] For individuals with SHCNs, some of these overarching principles into adult health care include

- "In whatever health care setting it is delivered, services need to be appropriate for both chronologic age and developmental attainment;
- Adolescents and young adults with chronic conditions share many of the same health issues and concerns as their peers. Thus, transitional health programs should be prepared to address common concerns of young people, including growth and development, sexuality, mood and other mental health disorders, substance use, and other health-promoting and health-damaging behaviors;
- Many adolescents with chronic conditions are at higher risk than peers for unnecessary dependency, developmental difficulties, and psychosocial delay. A successful transition to adult health care may help prevent this by enhancing autonomy, increasing a sense of personal responsibility, and facilitating self-reliance;
- Transition programs should be flexible enough to meet the needs of a wide range of young people, health conditions, and circumstances. The actual transfer of care should be individualized to meet the specific needs of young people and their families;
- HCT is most successful when there is a designated professional who, together with the patient and family, takes responsibility for the process. Each patient and family should have a coordinator and advocate who help to facilitate and streamline their transition experience."[3]

Other principles cited in the HCT literature that are pertinent not only for youth with SHCNs but also for those without medical and/or special needs include

- Interdisciplinary shared responsibilities, care-coordination, and effective communication between the pediatric and adult health care teams;
- Recognition that social determinants of health, cultural beliefs, transition readiness, presence of medical and/or dental homes, insurance coverage, gender, sexual orientation, race, as well as education and socioeconomic status have an influence on HCT;
- Efforts to achieve health equity and eliminate health care disparities;
- Recognition of patients' individual needs, differences, and vulnerabilities;
- Early discussion and implementation of a systematic HCT planning into adult health care;
- When possible, emphasis on the importance of patients' independence, self-management, autonomy, decision-making regarding their own health, as well as continuous use of health care;

- When available, caregivers' support and engagement from the beginning of the HCT process.[7,8,13,14]

Barriers to Successful Transitions

Although the definition, goals, and principles proposed for HCT seem reasonable, there are several barriers preventing a successful transition.[4–9,15,27] While these barriers are encountered by healthy individuals, they present an even greater challenge for those with chronic diseases and SHCNs.[4,5,9] The medical literature on the HCT of patients with chronic diseases and SHCNs is more extensive than the dental literature; however, similar trends have been found in both fields.

Shortage of adult dental care providers

There is an overall consensus in the literature that a significant barrier to successful HCT for young adults with SHCNs is a shortage of general dentists who are willing and able to provide dental care for individuals with SHCNs.[5,8,10,16,27–29] A national survey revealed that only 10% of general dentists in the US reported seeing children with SHCNs either "very often" or "often."[27] Over 60% of the respondents selected "patient behavior" as the greatest barrier to their willingness to provide care for these children, and over 45% reported the level of the patient's disability as a barrier to treating this population. In another national survey, pediatric dentists in both private practice and academics cited the availability of general dentists and specialists as the major barrier to HCT for adolescents with SHCNs.[5] Lack of adequate training and insufficient exposure to treating individuals with SHCNs during dental school are among the many reasons general dentists reported for not feeling comfortable and capable treating this population.[27,30,31] Pediatric dentistry is considered an "age-defined specialty that provides both primary and comprehensive preventive and therapeutic oral health care for infants and children through adolescence, including those with SHCNs."[32] However, owing to a shortage of general dentists who accept adult patients with SHCNs, pediatric dentists are often called upon to provide care for these individuals because they are trained in behavior management and the care of those who are medically and developmentally compromised. On the one hand, general dentists do not feel adequately trained and qualified to manage the behavior and complex needs of patients with SHCNs. On the other hand, pediatric dentists do not feel adequately trained and qualified to provide the optimal adult care that patients with SHCNs may require, especially for dental procedures that fall outside the scope of their training.

Patient and caregiver characteristics

Results from the 2005 to 2006 national survey that addressed HCT planning for children with SHCNs showed significant disparities in race/ethnicity and socioeconomic status among the individuals with SHCNs who were surveyed.[4] Adolescents who were Hispanic and non-Hispanic Black, living in non–English-speaking and low-income households, were less likely to achieve transition successfully.[4] The same survey conducted in 2009 to 2010 revealed that adolescents (aged 12–17 years) whose special needs consistently affected their daily lives were half as likely to receive services for transitioning to an adult medical care system than those whose special needs did not affect their daily activities (25.5% vs 52.0%).[33] The same pattern was observed for adolescents living in poverty when compared to those in the highest income households (25.4% vs 52.2%). A more recent national survey (2016–2017) reported that fewer than 20% of adolescents diagnosed with behavioral, developmental, and/or mental disorders, particularly those with autism spectrum disorder, received appropriate and successful services to assist with transitioning to adult medical care.[17]

Non-English speakers are less likely to have discussions with clinicians about transition, use dental care, and achieve satisfactory HCT.[4] Adolescents with SHCNs whose parents have low education levels also are known to face barriers to HCT.[12] These studies[4,12,17,33] identified a subset of vulnerable individuals with SHCNs who do not meet the requirements for HCT. Individuals with SHCNs who are least likely to receive HCT services are those from low-income and minority groups, who have low-educated parents, and who present with functional limitations and/or medical conditions associated with mental, behavioral, and/or developmental disorders. As a result, they do not secure needed medical and oral health care as they move into adulthood. Therefore, to ensure successful HCT, it is crucial to give priority to this population and provide the necessary support to help them and their families navigate the complex health system.

A study[9] using data from 2 national surveys examined the association between having a medical care transition plan and dental care use during the transition from adolescence to adulthood. It also identified factors that influence dental care use for individuals with SHCNs, both with and without functional limitations; that is, ability to participate in daily activities.[9] HCT was defined as a process for adolescents with SHCNs that included having a discussion with the primary care provider on "how health needs might change with age" and ever developing a transition plan.[9] Results showed that having an HCT plan was a "key determinant of dental care use" only for individuals with SHCNs who did not present with any functional limitation. Regardless of the individual's functional limitation status, a higher family income and adequate medical care insurance were the 2 factors consistently associated with a greater likelihood of dental care use. However, having an HCT plan in place is not enough to guarantee dental care use among individuals with SHCNs, especially for those with functional limitations.[9] Financial limitations are problematic for adults with SHCNs because most are covered by public insurance programs, with little to no coverage for dental services. Without private insurance and/or the financial means necessary to pay for out-of-pocket dental expenses not covered by public insurance, the utilization of dental care within this population is potentially reduced. In addition, it is important to recognize that individuals with SHCNs have many other expensive health care needs that take priority over dental care.[12]

An important obstacle to a successful HCT is the difficulty of breaking the bond and long-lasting relationship with a pediatric health care provider.[5,11,12,14] Patients and their families perceive that pediatric providers know their needs well, are more patient- than dental-focused, and have a more welcoming and cheerful clinic atmosphere.[11] Negative beliefs about adult health care include, but are not limited to, the idea that adult providers do not listen to or value caregivers' knowledge about their adolescents' SHCNs. In addition, there is a fear of the unknown when transitioning to a new adult care system, with patients and caregivers anticipating differences between pediatric and adult therapy recommendations.[14] Caregivers of and patients with more complex medical and developmental needs are reported to not mind continued care by pediatric dentists into adulthood, whereas more independent and self-sufficient adolescents report feeling "out of place or infantilized" in a pediatric setting and are more likely to welcome the transition to an adult dentist.[11] Caregivers of Medicaid-enrolled adolescents with SHCNs cite difficulties in finding general dentists who accept public insurance programs and changes in insurance benefits, from childhood to adulthood, as reasons to continue care at their "home" pediatric dentist office.[11]

Many adolescents with SHCNs expect the transition into the adult care system to be supported and facilitated by their families, medical, and/or dental teams.[11] Those with unstable living conditions who lack the support of a caregiver, family, or group home system are at increased risk of not only failing to transition but also not having appropriate access to medical and dental care.[12,14] Although pediatric dentists are reported to help their adolescent patients with and without SHCNs transition into the adult care system,[5] there is still a lack of general dentists and specialists who accept patients with SHCNs with behavioral and complex needs, as well as those with public insurance programs. Moreover, there is a lack of readiness on the part of patients and caregivers to make the transition. These factors contribute to some patients with SHCNs over the age of 21 years continuing to rely on pediatric dentists for their dental care.

Providers' characteristics

An important consideration that prevents pediatric dentists from transitioning adolescent patients with SHCNs into adult care is that most of these patients are covered by public dental insurance, which is often not accepted by many general dentists due to low reimbursement rates.[28,29] When pediatric and general dentists were interviewed about the transition for adolescents with SHCNs, most agreed that the transition would facilitate continuity of care and establishing a stable dental home for the patient.[10] The most common barriers for a successful transition, reported by both pediatric and general dentists, were a shortage of qualified general dentists who are "comfortable, experienced, and willing" to provide dental care for individuals with SHCNs and low dental reimbursement by public insurance programs.[10] These findings were consistent with those from other studies.[5,8,16,27–29] As with dentists, pediatric and adult physicians report similar obstacles to HCT, with the greatest difficulty being the transition of patients with more complex medical needs.[18] In addition, both medical and dental providers report other challenges, including lack of communication and coordination between providers, differences in styles between pediatric and adult practices, appropriate reimbursement, and availability of office staff to dedicate time and effort to help patients and their families with the transition process.[5,8,14,16]

Models of Health Care Transitions

Although a policy on "Transitioning from a Pediatric-Centered to an Adult-Centered Dental Home for Individuals with Special Health Care Needs" was adopted by the American Academy of Pediatric Dentistry in 2011,[16] a recent literature review demonstrates that there is minimal knowledge, evidence, and research to guide the transition from a pediatric to an adult dental care system for these patients.[17]

The medical field is ahead of dentistry in terms of developing, implementing, and testing HCT models. After the release of a clinical report on HCT in 2011,[15] developed in collaboration with the American Academy of Pediatrics, the American Academy of Family Physicians, and the American College of Physicians, a structured clinical approach, called "Six Core Elements of Health Care Transition," was developed to assist pediatric, family, and internal medicine physicians transitioning patients with and without special needs to an adult-centered care system.[16] An updated version of this approach was developed in 2020, after the original model was tested in different clinical settings (ie, rural, suburban, urban, and academic sites) and later reviewed by clinicians, nurses, social workers, family navigators, public health experts, patients, and caregivers.[18] This transition approach is divided into 6 timely stages that initiate early in adolescence and continue into young adulthood: "(1) Policy/Guide (age 12–14 years): develop, discuss, and share transition and care policy-guide; (2) Tracking and Monitoring (age 14–18 years): track progress using a flow sheet registry; (3) Readiness (age 14–18 years): assess self-care skills and offer education on identified needs; (4) planning (age 14–18 years): develop HCT plan with medical summary; (5) Transfer of Care (age 18–21 years): transfer to adult-centered care and to an adult practice; and (6) Transition Completion (age 18–23 years): confirm completion and elicit consumer feedback."[18] Additional considerations for individuals with SHCNs are implemented in the "Six Core Elements of Health Care Transition" to address their specific needs.[6,18] These special considerations include, but are not limited to, assessment of the patient's degree of independence, decision-making, and self-advocacy; care coordination and comanagement between primary care providers and specialists; and written action-oriented care plans, as well as plans to address issues related to family/caregiver support, informed consent, guardianship or power of attorney, and insurance coverage.[6,18]

RECOMMENDATIONS

Dentistry is significantly lagging when it comes to providing accessible and adequate dental care for individuals with SHCNs, as well as successfully transitioning this population from a pediatric- to an adult-centered dental care system. Certainly, as illustrated in **Fig. 1**, it will take a support system of concurring elements to nurture an environment conducive to successful transition. Federal and state public insurance programs (ie, Medicaid) need to extend benefits and services received in childhood throughout adolescence and adulthood for these individuals, as well as reimburse practitioners for the transitional process. General dentists make up the majority in the dental workforce[34]; therefore, they must be adequately trained during dental school or specialty trainings and/or through continuing education courses to assume the duty of caring for patients with SHCNs aging out of pediatrics.[28,29] There is an urgent need to change the dental curriculum to allow students to not only "assess the treatment needs of patients with special needs" but more importantly to obtain meaningful clinical experiences in treating individuals with SHCNs of all ages.[28,29] Efforts to recognize special care dentistry as a specialty in the US should continue, in an attempt to increase the number of qualified dentists that can treat individuals with SHCNs and decrease disparities within this population.[28,29] General dentists

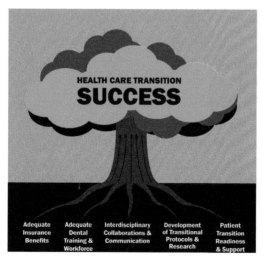

Fig. 1. Illustration of a support system of concurring elements needed to ensure successful transition from a pediatric- to an adult-centered dental care system.

should consider being the dental home for children with SHCNs, preferably no later than 12 months of age. This would allow general dentists to establish a relationship with the patient and their family early in life, become familiar with the child's special needs, and learn how to deal with potential challenges as the child grows older. Interdisciplinary collaborations among providers from different professional organizations, with expertize and/or training in the care of individuals with SHCNs (ie, general practice, advanced education in general dentistry, geriatric dentistry, pediatric dentistry, special care dentistry, dental public health) are needed to develop transitional policies and protocols that address the dental, medical, behavioral, and socioeconomic needs of adolescents ready to transition from pediatrics. Moreover, interdisciplinary communication and teamwork are crucial for the success of HCT. The referring dentist should identify and establish partnerships with those in their community who are willing to treat patients with SHCNs and subsequently provide support to the referred dentist by sharing detailed information about the patient's specific needs and comanaging care until the transition is finalized. The use of teledentistry as a means to provide guidance through teleconsultations may also be beneficial for all parties involved in the transition process.[35] Researchers in the field are called to examine the impact that dental transition protocols and strategies have on long-term oral health outcomes and barriers to accessing dental care within the SHCN population. Finally, it is crucial to evaluate the patient and their caregiver readiness to transition and provide them with the education and support necessary for a successful HCT.

The US dental care system is not equipped to provide dental care for individuals with SHCNs, regardless of their age.[34] Such an unacceptable, ongoing crisis calls for significant and necessary changes. There is still much that needs to be done and learned to ensure that individuals with SHCNs receive adequate dental care and successfully transition from a pediatric to an adult care system. In the meantime, it is important to target all high-risk populations at this critical stage of life who are less likely to access adequate oral health care and achieve satisfactory transition.

SUMMARY

1. Adequate dental training is needed to increase the number of qualified dentists that can treat individuals with SHCNs when they age out from pediatrics.
2. There is a paucity in the dental literature regarding transition policies and protocols from pediatrics-centered to adult-centered care for individuals with SHCNs.
3. There are significant disparities in race/ethnicity, socioeconomic status, and health status among individuals with SHCNs who do not achieve successful HCT.
4. Research is needed to evaluate transition protocols/strategies and assess their impact on oral health outcomes among individuals with SHCNs.

CLINICS CARE POINTS

- It is estimated that 90% of individuals with special health care needs (SHCN) and chronic conditions who require specialized medical and dental care live into adulthood. Therefore, it is important to successfully transition these individuals into the adult health care system to receive comprehensive care that is medically and developmentally appropriate for their age and complex needs.

- Individuals with SHCN who have successfully transitioned from a pediatric- to an adult-centered care are more likely to receive continuous care, which has the greatest positive impact on their long-term health outcomes.

- The planning and support for health care transition (HCT) should be initiated early and be part of the routine primary care for all adolescents, especially those with SHCN.

- Individuals with SHCN who are least likely to receive HCT services are those from low-income and minority groups, who have low-educated parents and present with functional limitations and/or medical conditions associated with mental, behavioral, and/or developmental disorders.

- Interdisciplinary collaborations, communication and teamwork are crucial for the success of HCT of individuals with SHCN from a pediatric- to an adult-care system.

ACKNOWLEDGMENT

The author would like to thank Jeanna Holmes from the University of Iowa Department of Pediatric Dentistry for the design of **Fig. 1**.

DISCLOSURE

The author has nothing to disclose.

REFERENCES

1. Blum RW, D Garell D, Hodgman CH, et al. Transition from child-centered to adult health-care systems for adolescents with chronic conditions. A position paper of the Society for Adolescent Medicine. J Adolesc Health 1993;14(7):570–6.
2. Blum RW. Introduction. Improving transition for adolescents with special health care needs from pediatric to adult-centered health care. Pediatrics 2003; 111(2):449.
3. Rosen DS, Blum RW, Britto M, et al. Transition to adult health care for adolescents and young adults with chronic conditions: position paper of the Society for Adolescent Medicine. J Adolesc Health 2003;33(4):309–11.
4. Lotstein DS, Ghandour R, Cash A, et al. Planning for health care transitions: results from the 2005-2006 national survey of children with special health care needs. Pediatrics 2009;123(1):e145–52.
5. Nowak AJ, Casamassimo PS, Slayton RL. Facilitating the transition of patients with special health care needs from pediatric to adult oral health care. J Am Dent Assoc 2010;141(11):1351–6.
6. Cooley WC, Sagerman PJ. Supporting the health care transition from adolescence to adulthood in the medical home. Pediatrics 2011;128(1):182–200.
7. McManus MA, Pollack LR, Cooley WC, et al. Current status of transition preparation among youth with special needs in the United States. Pediatrics 2013;131(6): 1090–7.
8. Borromeo GL, Bramante G, Betar D, et al. Transitioning of special needs paediatric patients to adult special needs dental services. Aust Dent 2014;59(3):360–5.
9. Chi DL. Medical care transition planning and dental care use for youth with special health care needs during the transition from adolescence to young adulthood: a preliminary explanatory model. Matern Child Health J 2014;18(4):778–88.
10. Bayarsaikhan Z, Cruz S, Neff J, et al. Transitioning from pediatric to adult dental care for adolescents with special health care needs: dentist perspectives–part two. Pediatr Dent 2015;37(5):447–51.
11. Cruz S, Neff J, Chi DL. Transitioning from pediatric to adult dental care for adolescents with special health care needs: adolescent and parent perspectives–part one. Pediatr Dent 2015;37(5):442–6.

12. Gray WN, Schaefer MR, Resmini-Rawlinson A, et al. Barriers to transition from pediatric to adult care: a systematic review. J Pediatr Psychol 2018;43(5):488–502.

13. Lebrun-Harris LA, McManus MA, Ilango SM, et al. Transition planning among US youth with and without special health care needs. Pediatrics 2018;142(4): e20180194.

14. White PH, Cooley WC. Supporting the health care transition from adolescence to adulthood in the medical home. Pediatrics 2018;142(5):e20182587.

15. American Academy of Pediatric Dentistry. Policy on transitioning from a pediatric-centered to an adult-centered dental home for individuals with special health care needs. The Reference Manual of Pediatric Dentistry. Chicago, IL: American Academy of Pediatric Dentistry; 2020. p. 152–5.

16. Chavis S, Canares G. The transition of patients with special health care needs from pediatric to adult-based dental care: a scoping review. Pediatr Dent 2020; 42(2):101–9.

17. Leeb RT, Danielson ML, Bitsko RH, et al. Support for transition from adolescent to adult health care among adolescents with and without mental, behavioral, and developmental disorders - United States, 2016-2017. MMWR Morb Mortal Wkly Rep 2020;69(34):1156–60.

18. White PH, Schmidt A, Shorr J, et al. Six core elements of health care transition™ 3.0. Washington, DC: Got Transition, The National Alliance to Advance Adolescent Health; 2020.

19. Zablotsky B, Black LI. Prevalence of children aged 3-17 years with developmental disabilities, by ubanicity: United States, 2015-2018. Natl Health Stat Rep 2020;(139):1–7.

20. Okoro CA, Hollis ND, Cyrus AC, et al. Prevalence of disabilities and health care access by disability status and type among adults - United States, 2016. MMWR Morb Mortal Wkly Rep 2018;67(32):882–7.

21. Chi DL. Oral health for US children with special health care needs. Pediatr Clin North Am 2018;65(5):981–93.

22. American Academy of Pediatric Dentistry. Definition of special health care needs. The Reference Manual of Pediatric Dentistry. Chicago, IL: American Academy of Pediatric Dentistry; 2020. p. 19.

23. Houtenville A, Rafal M. Annual report on people with disabilities in America. Durham, NH: University of New Hampshire, Institute on Disability; 2020.

24. Paul S, Rafal M, Houtenville A. Annual disability statistics supplement. Durham, NH: University of New Hampshire, Institute on Disability; 2020.

25. Perrin JM, Bloom SR, Gortmaker SL. The increase of childhood chronic conditions in the United States. JAMA 2007;297(24):2755–9.

26. Young NAE. Childhood disability in the United States: 2019 ACSBR-006. Washington, DC: American Community Survey Briefs, U.S. Census Bureau; 2021.

27. Casamassimo PS, Seale NS, Ruehs K. General dentists' perceptions of educational and treatment issues affecting access to care for children with special health care needs. J Dent Educ 2004;68(1):23–8.

28. Waldman HB, Ackerman MB, Perlman SP. Increasing use of dental services by children, but many are unable to secure needed care. J Clin Pediatr Dent 2014;39(1):9–11.

29. Waldman HB, Rader R, Sulkes S, et al. Pediatric dentistry specialty as part of a longer continuum of care: a commentary. J Clin Pediatr Dent 2016;40(5):341–4.

30. Dao LP, Zwetchkenbaum S, Inglehart MR. General dentists and special needs patients: does dental education matter? J Dent Educ 2005;69(10):1107–15.

31. Hicks J, Vishwanat L, Perry M, et al. SCDA task force on a special care dentistry residency. Spec Care Dentist 2016;36(4):201–12.
32. American Academy of Pediatric Dentistry. Definitions and scope of pediatric dentistry. The Reference Manual of Pediatric Dentistry. Chicago, IL: American Academy of Pediatric Dentistry; 2021. p. 7–9.
33. U.S. Department of Health and Human Services, Health Resources and Services Administration, Maternal and Child Health Bureau. The national survey of children with special health care needs Chartbook 2009–2010. Rockville, Maryland: U.S. Department of Health and Human Services; 2013.
34. Kerins C, Casamassimo PS, Ciesla D, et al. A preliminary analysis of the US dental health care system's capacity to treat children with special health care needs. Pediatr Dent 2011;33(2):107–12.
35. Alabdullah JH, Daniel SJ. A systematic review on the validity of teledentistry. Telemed J E Health 2018;24(8):639–48.

Adolescent Dental Fear and Anxiety
Background, Assessment, and Nonpharmacologic Behavior Guidance

Janice A. Townsend, DDS, MS[a,b,]*, Cameron L. Randall, PhD[c]

KEYWORDS

- Adolescents • Behavior guidance • Dental fear • Dental anxiety
- Special health care needs • COVID-19

KEY POINTS

- Adolescence is a critically important developmental stage and a time of vulnerability for the acquisition of dental fear and/or anxiety.
- Evidence-based tools, such as the Modified Dental Anxiety Scale (MDAS), should be used to assess dental fear and anxiety.
- Nonpharmacologic techniques from cognitive-behavior therapy, such as diaphragmatic breathing, distraction, and systematic desensitization, are effective in this age group.
- Dental professionals should be comfortable in enlisting behavioral health professionals as allies in care for patients with severe dental fear, anxiety, or phobia.

INTRODUCTION

Dental caries is the most common disease of childhood and adolescence[1] and yet almost all dental treatment in the United States is performed without sedation or general anesthesia.[2] In addition to providing competent clinical care, dentists must also use techniques to shape behavior, allay anxiety, and promote coping. This process has traditionally been called behavior management, where the dentist focuses on obtaining cooperation to complete the needed procedures regardless of long-term effects.[3] A more contemporary approach is behavior guidance, where the dentist acts as a coach to promote coping and lifelong positive views of dentistry.[4]

The authors have nothing to disclose.
[a] Department of Dentistry, Nationwide Children's Hospital, 700 Children's Drive, LA Suite 5A, Columbus, OH 43205, USA; [b] Division of Pediatric Dentistry, The Ohio State University, Columbus, OH, USA; [c] Department of Oral Health Sciences, University of Washington School of Dentistry, 1959 NE Pacific Street, Box 357475, Seattle, WA 98195, USA
* Corresponding author. 700 Children's Drive, LA Suite 5A, Columbus, OH 43205.
E-mail address: Janice.Townsend@nationwidechildrens.org

Dent Clin N Am 65 (2021) 731–751
https://doi.org/10.1016/j.cden.2021.07.002
dental.theclinics.com

The literature on behavior guidance in dentistry has focused primarily on promoting cooperation with preschool-aged or school-aged patients. Even within this body of literature there are few techniques that are clearly supported by evidence to be superior to others.[5,6] With populations less frequently studied, such as adolescents, evidence supporting different interventions is more scarce, despite it being a critical time for acquisition or remission of dental fear.[7] This article reviews salient features of adolescent development in conjunction with conceptual issues related to dental fear, anxiety, and phobia. It reviews nonpharmacologic strategies to improve acceptance of dental treatment that can be provided by dental teams as well as guidance about when to involve mental health professionals (further guidance on pharmacologic management can be found in the Matthew Cooke and Thomas Tanbonliong's article, "Sedation and Anesthesia for the Adolescent Dental Patient," in this issue).

DEVELOPMENTAL CONSIDERATIONS FOR BEHAVIOR GUIDANCE IN ADOLESCENCE

Adolescence is a critically important developmental stage of transition from childhood to adulthood. The American Academy of Pediatrics has outlined numerous aspects of, and health challenges encountered during, this developmental stage, describing the needs of individuals 11 to 21 years old as "unique."[8] Several defining characteristics of adolescence have important implications for interactions with adolescent dental patients and also have implications for these young people's oral health–related behaviors and experiences.

In addition to physiologic changes (namely puberty), adolescence involves other significant biological as well as psychosocial changes. Ongoing brain development is experienced throughout adolescence.[9] Changes in the regions of the brain that regulate impulse control and changes in the brain's reward system increase not only risk-taking behavior but also the intensity of adolescents' response to emotionally loaded situations.[8] This observation is especially true in early and middle adolescence, with capacity for emotion regulation increasing across adolescence.[10] These changes and their effects are a normal part of development, and conceptualizations of adolescence as a period of disturbance and problem behavior have long been debunked by developmental scientists.[11] That is, the supposed problems most adolescents experience typically are transitory, part of the process of development, and resolved by adulthood. However, these changes may result in emotional sequelae that have relevance to adolescents' experience of potentially emotionally loaded dental encounters. Thus, emotionality should be considered by dental clinicians. Beginning in early adolescence and coinciding with white matter increases, noteworthy and often fairly rapid improvements in reasoning, information processing, and complex cognitive abilities are typical.[10,12] The result of these changes is increased abstract, multidimensional, and planned thinking as well as adaptive behavior.[8,10] Adverse childhood experiences can affect various aspects of this cognitive development.[13]

Adolescents' social development is just as profound as their cognitive development. It is true that the adolescent-parent relationship goes through significant transformations during adolescence; however, this transformation is rarely as negative and riddled with alienation and rebellion as is often portrayed in popular culture.[14] More typical adolescent-parent relationship changes include a movement from hierarchical to egalitarian relationships through a process that involves less intense, but still complicated and sometimes difficult, conflict, distancing, and separation.[14–16] This process is normal and, compared with no conflict or frequent conflict, some conflict with parents is linked to better adjustment.[14,17] Culture, economic security, structural changes (eg, divorce), and parenting styles can affect this process.[14] As the adolescent-parent relationship transforms, adolescents simultaneously spend increasing time alone and with friends.[18] Contrary to some portrayals of peer influences on adolescents as potentially largely negative, most adolescent-peer relationships are characterized by increasing closeness, disclosing, and support.[19] However, adolescent-peer relationships can be complicated, particularly when considering the larger social context, and this may result in interpersonal difficulty and emotional distress.[14] Note that the influence of peers on adolescents can be both positive and negative and that the influence is less often coercive and more often the product of admiration and respect.[11] This social development in adolescence is mediated by brain and cognitive development.[20]

A defining feature of adolescence is increasing independence. Refinement of the social self and a deepening and cementing of the adolescents' identity occur across adolescence.[21] Beginning in early adolescence, people's self-concept becomes more abstract and nuanced.[11] Although there is often some instability during middle adolescence, by late adolescence most people have developed an organized sense of self.[22] Along with changing parent and peer relationships, this results in an identity, beliefs, and behaviors that are unique to the individual and that can persist well into adulthood. An adolescent's transition to independence has implications for health behaviors, including the future patterns of health that are established during this critical period.[23–26] As such, the National Institute of Dental and Craniofacial Research importantly suggests that healthy behaviors and health promotion during adolescence can benefit oral and overall health into adulthood.[27] Likewise, adolescents' experiences with health care and the coping skills they develop to manage potential distress during health care visits can have lifetime influence.

FEAR, ANXIETY, AND PHOBIA: CONCEPTUAL ISSUES

Understanding dental care–related fear, anxiety, and phobia as the complex, multifactorial, and highly individualized experiences they are is essential to applying the appropriate behavior guidance techniques and other strategies for effective management. Although much of what is known about fear, anxiety, and phobia (including that related to dental care) is universal across the lifespan, some of the aforementioned developmental considerations unique to adolescence are helpful for fully appreciating the emotional experience and its consequences. Within the dental care–related fear and anxiety literature, limited specialized attention has been paid to adolescents, but certain developmental considerations can be mapped onto what is known.

Although overlapping and often described interchangeably, dental care–related fear, anxiety, and phobia represent 3 distinct emotional and behavioral phenomena.[28–30] Briefly, fear is an immediate emotional response to stimuli perceived to be threatening and is often characterized by physiologic arousal (ie, sympathetic responding or panic symptoms), reports of apprehension, and avoidance behavior.[30–32] This response is distinguished from anxiety, which often also involves physiologic responsivity, though frequently less robust, and typically is much more cognitively involved, characterized by more pronounced negative thoughts and worries about possible or future encounters with stimuli perceived to be threatening.[30–32] In other words, fear is the in-the-moment emotional response to potentially dangerous situations and anxiety is what occurs distally in time with respect to the situation. Most succinctly, phobia describes an impairing and emotionally distressing experience wherein avoidance resulting from fear and/or anxiety is so significant that it affects functioning and health (eg, consistent excessive delaying of dental treatment because of fear/anxiety that leads to unmet treatment needs, pain, and poorer quality of life).[32,33] Phobias typically are diagnosed by a mental health professional.

Although most patients with fears and anxieties about dental treatment experience both emotions, it is often the case that patients experience one more than the other.[32] Appreciating the distinction is thus helpful in selecting the most appropriate behavior guidance techniques and other strategies for management. Pediatric providers may find it especially useful to distinguish between fear and anxiety in adolescents. Because they have increasingly developed abstract thinking skills and higher-level cognitive processes as they age, they may be more likely to present with worry or rumination (ie, anxiety). Moreover, they may be experiencing this emotional reaction to dentistry for the first time. Helping these patients to manage pretreatment anxiety (and not just helping them cope with in-the-moment distress during a dental visit) thus may be especially useful.

Also critical to understanding dental care–related fear and anxiety is appreciating the patient's experience of the phenomena occurs along a continuum.[30] On 1 end of the continuum is a complete absence of fear and anxiety; on the other is phobia, with significant emotional distress and excessive or complete avoidance of dental stimuli. Some degree of fear and anxiety about dental treatment might be expected and considered normal, in part because there are indeed aspects of dental care that are unpleasant or uncomfortable at times (eg, potential for pain, feeling closed in, perceiving a loss of control), or at least have the potential to be. Between the normal range and phobic levels, a patient can experience increasingly distressing fear and anxiety associated with increasing behavior disruptions and avoidance or attempts at avoidance.[33] Patients historically were thought of as being either fearful or not fearful of dental treatment; but contemporary research has revealed that the emotional experience is dimensional and involves a range of possible intensity and impact.[32] Given adolescents' abstract thinking skills, including more advanced numeracy, more nuanced assessment of fear and anxiety intensity is possible compared with children. Such assessment allows for the provision of more person-centered care that addresses the individualized nature of emotional experiences across the entire gradient.

The causes of dental care–related fear and anxiety are many and the influences that maintain or perpetuate fear, anxiety, and the behavioral sequelae are complex. A more specific review of the dental literature regarding all the causes of dental care–related fear, anxiety, and phobia is included later but an exhaustive review is beyond the scope of this article; instead, readers are directed to a few reviews, book chapters, and books.[32–37] Briefly, numerous causal mechanisms and predisposing factors have been identified, including learning (especially associative learning; ie, conditioning), social learning (including intergenerational transmission), cognitive processes (ie, thoughts), temperament and personality, pain sensitivity and pain perception, and distress tolerance.[32,33] Three of these causal pathways/factors have particular relevance to adolescents' experience of dental care–related fear and anxiety.

First, conditioned fear or anxiety accounts for a potentially large proportion of the dental care–related fear and anxiety experience.[33,38,39] In such a situation, patients who have painful or otherwise negative experiences in the dental setting associate the pain or distressing physical sensations with dental stimuli, such as the process of having a bib secured around the neck, the sight of a masked clinician, the sound of a drill, or the characteristic smell of the operatory. Subsequently, these patients can experience distress when they encounter those same stimuli, even in the absence of pain or discomfort, and they may show behavior management problems or avoid dental care to avoid the distress. Fear can be caused in this manner at any age, but it is known to be common and more frequent among younger people.[40,41] For instance, of adults who report dental care–related fear, nearly one-quarter endorse onset in adolescence (and more than half in childhood), with prior painful or otherwise negative experiences cited as the most common cause.[42] Similarly, approximately 35% of children aged 6 to 14 years report having experienced pain during dental care.[43] In addition to using good pain control strategies, it may be particularly helpful to adolescents to explain clinical procedures and the stimuli encountered, because they are cognitively able to use this information to cope or make sense of what otherwise might be perceived as more threatening than it actually is.

Second, social learning can account for fears and anxieties about dental treatment when a person has not previously had a painful or negative experience with dentistry.[32–34] That is, fear and anxiety can be caused by communication or observational learning. In these cases, someone may hear about an aversive dental experience from a parent, friend, or other source (eg, mass entertainment or media outlets) or may witness someone else's pain or fear reaction to dental stimuli.[34,44] Generalized or specific worries about dental treatment–related stimuli or fear reactions in the dental setting can follow. Considering age-related social development, adolescents' primary source of information about dental stimuli as threatening may shift from parents to peers, and so it may be increasingly appropriate to ask questions such as, "What have you heard from your friends about this?" in order to fully understand the fear and anxiety experience. Note that the prevalence of this fear acquisition pathway likely is much lower than for direct conditioning and the evidence for this cause much less robust.[33]

Third, for children, adolescents, and adults, cognitive factors can play a role in the development and maintenance of dental care–related fear and anxiety.[32,33,37] People's perceptions of themselves in relation to the dental setting, and their thoughts about dental stimuli and self-efficacy related to coping, can facilitate fear and anxiety acquisition (or can be protective).[33] Several cognitive factors influence fear, anxiety, behavior, and symptom perception in the context of dentistry, such as misperceptions and misappraisal of threat/risk (eg, cognitive distortions including catastrophizing), rumination about and overestimation of pain, worries about lack of control, beliefs about dentistry and dentists, and trust.[37,45–48] Moreover, Armfield[49] identified 4 specific categories of misperceptions strongly associated with dental care–related fear: dangerousness, disgustingness, uncontrollability, and unpredictability. Although data for adolescents, specifically, are limited, 1 study found that perceived lack of control was highly associated with greater levels of dental care–related fear.[50] Given the rapid cognitive development, increasing sense of self, and increasing independence that characterize adolescence, these cognitive factors may be especially important for understanding and intervening on adolescents' fear, anxiety, and associated behavior, certainly more so than for children.

DENTAL FEAR, ANXIETY, AND PHOBIA IN THE ADOLESCENT POPULATION

As previously stated, dental care–related fear and anxiety have multifactorial origins that include patient characteristics such as intelligence, general anxiety, temperament, and context with regard to past experiences, culture, and socioeconomic status.[36,51]

The prevalence of dental fear/anxiety varies between 10% and 29.3% depending on the instrument and geographic location used.[52] Conservatively, 1 adolescent out of 10 has a level of dental fear and or anxiety that is an impediment to dental care.[52] Studies from the United States have ranged from 20% to 29.6% and anxiety is higher compared with northern Europe.[52,53] This prevalence is likely an underestimate of the general population because studies in dental settings do not capture individuals with avoidance.[33]

Female sex is almost certainly a risk factor for increased risk of dental fear and anxiety. Studies conducted in diverse cultural populations identify women significantly more fearful then men,[52,54–65] although a minority of studies have not found a significant difference.[7,50,66] The relationship between anxiety and sex may be related to increasing age,[61] and age 14 years has been identified as a turning point when boys show higher acceptance of dental treatment than girls.[67]

It is unclear how much of the disparity in reporting of anxiety by sex is a true reflection of fear or caused by differential reporting. The acceptability of showing emotions that are considered weak is conditioned by gender in many cultures and may affect these data.[63] It is possible that women have been conditioned to communicate fear as part of the coping process, whereas vocalizing this anxiety may exacerbate fear of failure in men. When patients' reports of anxiety are compared with parental reports, girls report significantly more anxiety than boys, but the mothers' reports of children's anxiety do not differ.[68]

Studies suggest that women and men interpret dentist characteristics differently.[69] For men, perceived lack of control is more negatively experienced[50,69] and associated with fear and avoidance.[50] Perceived belittlement was also an important factor for men; whereas, women rated trust and communication as most important.[69] Knowledge of these general principles can help clinicians, but gender norms vary by culture and by individual so, when establishing rapport, dentists should inquire about dentists' characteristics that would make patients most comfortable.

Younger age is a risk factor for higher dental fear and anxiety across the span of childhood. Studies suggest that, within the ages that constitute the period of adolescence, younger individuals are still significantly more fearful than older ones,[54,66] although others have found that age is unrelated in this subgroup.[52,55,65] The relationship between age and dental fear and anxiety in the adolescent age group is undoubtedly related to experience, own or observed, with dental treatment.

Behavior management problems have been found to be more common in children with lower socioeconomic status, and lack of parental cohabitation is also a contributor.[51] For adolescents, lower socioeconomic status is likely a risk factor for dental fear and anxiety.[56,60,66] This relationship is probably the result of increased caries burden and poorer quality of dental experiences. However, the relationship between oral health and fear in adolescents is not necessarily straightforward. Higher acceptance of treatment has been found in adolescents with no dental needs compared with those needing dental care.[68] Others found dental caries was only related to dental fear in boys but not girls.[55] In addition, studies have found no relationship between caries[54,64] and gingival health in adolescents with or without dental fear.[64]

Regularity of care and pain experienced during dental visits is almost certainly more important than presence or absence of disease at a specific point in time.[70] Adolescents with regular dental care who can identify a family dentist have reported lower incidences of fear.[50] Dental fear and anxiety are typically lower in individuals that have not had invasive procedures, but, in children and adolescents who had received invasive treatment and attended the dentist regularly, fear was not increased compared with children without regular attendance.[71] Adolescents who only visit the dentist when in pain had more dental fear than adolescents who have more regular care patterns.[54] A history of painful treatment affects future dental care seeking, with individuals reporting previous pain during treatment 13 times more likely to report high dental fear and more than 15 times less likely to be willing to return to the dentist.[50,70] Episodic or irregular dental visiting patterns can be a predictor of increased dental anxiety,[7,54,56] and the association between irregular dental care and dental anxiety can set up a vicious cycle of painful treatment and avoidance behavior.[7]

It may be assumed that the irregularity of dental care may have originated from a negative dental experience, but adolescents who had never visited the dentist have indicated more fear than adolescents who had dental visits in some populations.[54] Thus other factors, such as fear of pain or blood injury/injection phobia, may be predictors.[72,73]

Although maternal transmission of dental fear and anxiety is more commonly discussed in preschool children, there is a significant positive correlation between parental and child fear showing that the home environment is influential even at this age in contributing to intergenerational transmission of fear.[59,61,65,72] In low-income children, indirect modeling was the most commonly reported pathway. Thus, these models, whether they be parents, siblings, or peers, are more influential than in higher-income counterparts.[60] Altogether, dental fear and anxiety are likely the result of a combination of factors, including initial fear, experience of dental treatments, experience of toothache, and dental fear in the family.[57]

Dental fear and anxiety are related to general fear and both internalizing and externalizing behavior problems.[36] Higher general fears are more likely to be associated with high levels of dental fear but the opposite is not true: most children with high dental anxiety have low general fear.[56] Similarly, adolescents with high state anxiety are almost 3 times more likely to report dental fear than children with low state anxiety, but trait anxiety had no relationship.[58] No difference has been found in general anxiety between children and adolescents referred because of poor cooperation and those referred for other reasons, but higher increased impulsivity and negative emotionality have been found.[51,74]

In 18-year-olds, dentally anxious individuals were more likely to have a psychological disorder, and this correlation was primarily associated with highly dentally anxious individuals. The related psychological disorders were conduct disorder, agoraphobia, social phobia, simple phobia, and alcohol disorders. Teens with comorbid dental anxiety and psychological disorders were more likely to maintain their anxiety over time.[75]

ASSESSMENT OF DENTAL ANXIETY, FEAR, AND PHOBIA

As with the treatment of dental disease or other health problems, the first step in the management of distressing or impairing emotional experiences such as fear or anxiety is assessment. Identifying patients with higher levels of dental care–related fear and anxiety, and understanding the individualized manifestations and consequences of the fear/anxiety, is critical for successful management.[37,76,77] Dental providers often rely on clinical judgment, nonsystematic observation of behavior, or informal conversations to determine whether a patient is fearful or anxious.[78–81] Such assessment practices may be highly variable between dental providers, and findings are mixed regarding the validity of providers' clinical judgment in the assessment of dental care–related fear and anxiety for children and adolescents.[79,82,83] However, informally assessing the degree and nature of an adolescent's dental care–related fear or anxiety may be a worthwhile starting point. For instance, it can be useful to ask patients about treatment-related worries, including querying which specific aspects of dental care cause the most apprehension. It can also be useful to ask whether dental visits have been emotionally difficult in the past. This informal assessment should be intended as a conversation starter, perhaps serving as a screener, and open-ended questions (ie, not yes-no questions) and validating responses should be used by the provider.[32] Given adolescents' increasing capacity for emotional expression and abstract thinking, dental providers can reasonably expect increasing utility of informal assessment with age.[10]

Especially if informal assessment is suggestive of dental care–related fear and anxiety, but even better as a matter of routine practice, dental providers should use evidence-based tools to assess fears and anxieties.[32,37,79,84] As with adults, self-report instruments are the most commonly used type of validated tool for measuring dental care–related fear and anxiety among children and adolescents.[33,85] Although some self-report instruments have been studied with children as young as 3 or 4 years old (eg, Modified Child Dental Anxiety Scale), there is concern about the validity of such rating scales for younger children because of cognitive demands and not-yet-developed abstract thinking skills.[86–90] However, adolescence represents a developmental period when self-report instruments, especially those that use continuous (eg, Likert-type) scales, have increasing validity and reliability that tracks with chronologic age and cognitive development.[88,91]

Several self-report measures of dental care–related fear and anxiety have been used with adolescents in research and/or clinical settings, with adolescent-specific validity and reliability data available for some. Perhaps the most commonly used measure for adolescents and adults alike is the Modified Dental Anxiety Scale (MDAS).[92] The MDAS is a 5-item questionnaire involving rating how severe people predict their reactions would be to potentially anxiety-provoking dental stimuli. The MDAS is widely used, in part because of its short administration time; validity and reliability are good, and the instrument has been used with adolescents.[79,93–95] The other frequently used measure for assessing dental care–related fear and anxiety is the Dental Fear Survey (DFS).[96] The DFS is a 20-item questionnaire that quantifies fear and anxiety about dental treatment in 3 domains (ie, subscales): behavioral avoidance, physiologic responses, and fear of specific stimuli. Many studies provide evidence of validity and reliability.[97,98] The DFS has shown validity and utility in adolescent samples.[72,84] Because of its length, the DFS is more often used in research applications than in regular clinical practice; however, use of longer questionnaires may be preferred given that shorter questionnaires are critiqued for having limited focus.[84] One instrument, the Adolescents' Fear of Dental Treatment Cognitive Inventory, was developed specifically for use with adolescents.[99] Good validity and reliability were observed in the development study, although the instrument focuses only on cognitive aspects (and not physiologic or behavioral aspects) of fear and has not been used in subsequent studies, so the utility remains uncertain.[94] Numerous other instruments have been developed for use with adults and, although not yet validated for adolescents, may be still appropriate for adolescent patients (see Armfield[49] and Newton and Buck[94] for reviews). In addition, several instruments designed and validated specifically for use with children may be appropriate for use with younger adolescents or adolescents with developmental disabilities, language difficulties, or other special health care needs. Such instruments include the Children's Fear Survey Schedule Dental Subscale, the Modified Child Dental Anxiety Scale, and the Facial Image Scale[90,96,100–103]; see Porritt and colleagues,[84] Seligman and colleagues,[33] and Yon and colleagues[85] for reviews. Clinicians may also find utility in single-item instruments, most appropriately for use as screening tools. There are 2: the omnibus item of the DFS (question number 20) and the Dental Anxiety Question.[96,104] Most of the instruments described here, including the MDAS and DFS, have been translated into many languages.

With information gathered from a quality assessment, dental providers can tailor management approaches to the individualized presentation of fear and anxiety for any patient. For instance, behavior guidance techniques can be matched to the patient for effective management when the provider knows whether distress is experienced before treatment, during treatment, or both; whether distress is experienced physiologically in the form of panic symptoms or cognitively in the form of worry and catastrophic thinking; which dental stimuli cause the strongest fear or anxiety reactions (or whether the fear or anxiety is experienced more generally); and the extent to which someone is fearful or anxious (ie, where they are on the continuum and the degree of impact).

BEHAVIOR GUIDANCE TECHNIQUES FOR MANAGING DENTAL FEAR, ANXIETY, AND PHOBIA IN ADOLESCENCE

There are numerous effective behavior guidance techniques for managing dental care–related anxiety, fear, and phobia. Selection of techniques should be based on characteristics of the fear, anxiety, or phobia (drawing on a thorough, evidence-based assessment), characteristics of the dental treatment to be completed, the patient's developmental stage, and patient and/or caregiver preferences.[32,79] However, patient finances and access to behavioral health resources may affect some treatment options. Many of the most effective approaches for managing adolescent dental care–related fear and anxiety are the same as would be used when treating children or adults; however, some techniques may be particularly relevant when working with adolescents. These techniques are noted here as part of an overview of behavior guidance techniques, which are generally ordered from least to most intensive. Dental providers should appreciate that, in many cases, it is advisable to use more than 1 technique in any given clinical encounter.[32,37]

Good communication is the cornerstone of building trust and rapport.[79] For fearful or anxious patients, especially those with lower levels of fear/anxiety, use of basic counseling skills can go a long way to mitigate distress. First, asking about possible dental care–related fear or anxiety on intake forms or in the first encounter with patients can communicate sensitivity and often is validating for patients.[32] Focusing on patients' concerns and expectations in a direct manner is helpful.[37] The best way to engage in this communication is through active listening, including use of open-ended questions whenever possible, offering reflective statements in response to patients' answers, validating patients' emotions (vs simply providing reassurance, even if well intended), maintaining eye contact as much as possible when talking with patients, and monitoring tone for appropriateness.[32,105–107] The provision of information (sometimes referred to as patient education or psychoeducation) is another communication technique that can be helpful for preventing and managing distress associated with dental care–related fear and anxiety. Information about procedures can clarify uncertainties, dispel myths, and set expectations, all of which afford patients a sense of predictability.[79] Note that patients have differing preferences about the amount and type of information to be shared.[37,102] For some patients, too much information about the treatment plan or a particular procedure can exacerbate fear and anxiety; for others, detailed information can significantly allay fears and anxieties. It is advisable to ask patients whether they would find information distressing or reassuring, and, compared with younger people, many adolescents are able to answer this question to help guide the approach. Patients may also benefit from receipt of information about fear and anxiety, specifically. Understanding the basic conceptual issues described earlier, especially if delivered in a developmentally appropriate way, can help patients make sense of their emotional experiences, which can be reassuring and therapeutic,[103] particularly for adolescents because they are rapidly developing emotionally.

Because dental care–related fear and anxiety are strongly linked to perceived lack of control, especially among adolescents, behavior guidance techniques that offer control to patients are worthwhile.[50,108,109] Considering the provision of information, 1 way to offer a sense of control is to ask for permission before sharing details about a procedure or the nature of fear/anxiety (eg, "Is it okay with you if I share some information about the kinds of worries people your age have about dental treatment?").[110] Another commonly used approach for providing perceived control (and predictability) is using the tell-show-do technique. The American Academy of Pediatric Dentistry (AAPD) recommends offering a developmentally appropriate description of the procedures to be completed (ie, tell), a demonstration of the various aspects of the procedures (ie, show), and completion of the procedures in a way that does not deviate from the preceding description and demonstration.[4] Other techniques for providing control include planned regular (and dentist-initiated) rest breaks and patient-controlled signaling for break requests (see Armfield and Heaton[79] for detailed descriptions).[4,79] Consistency in the use and follow-through of these techniques is essential for building trust and managing and preventing fear/anxiety.[32,37] Asking adolescent patients what has been helpful for reducing fear or anxiety in the past, perhaps even before the dental provider offers any suggestions, or asking adolescent patients to teach a skill or direct its use may also engender feelings of control. Adolescence is a time of rapidly increasing understanding and exertion of autonomy, and so it is important to remember that issues of control may be particularly important for these patients.

Dental providers can minimize environmental triggers of dental care–related fear and anxiety by using stimulus control.[32] For instance, keeping fear-inducing stimuli (eg, syringe, handpiece) out of sight can help prevent distress. For some patients, seeing the syringe, including assembly, may allay anxiety. This technique is usually a last resort before instituting pharmacologic measures, but it has been successful for select cases. For patients who have previously had frightening injection experiences, using alternatives such as computer-controlled local anesthetic devices may help distinguish past experiences from potentially painless ones. However, even with the most experienced, skilled, and compassionate clinicians, dental treatment is potentially stressful for many patients. Several behavior guidance techniques drawn from cognitive-behavior therapy are useful in the management of this stress. First, diaphragmatic breathing can be efficiently taught to and practiced by adolescents with good effect, and it is likely to be more effective with this age group than for younger children.[111] Slow breaths are incompatible with the sympathetic (ie, fight-or flight) response that characterizes fear and anxiety, and thus induce relaxation, reducing fear/anxiety in the dental setting.[37,112] Second, distraction can reorient attention away from stimuli perceived to be threating to prevent fear/anxiety or induce relaxation.[37,79] As a general rule, more immersive distraction techniques are more effective. Studies have shown excellent benefit from various forms of distraction (eg, imagery, music, television, virtual reality) in the dental setting and especially for pediatric patients, including younger adolescents.[4,105,113,114] Third, given their cognitive development, adolescents may find more benefit than younger pediatric patients in cognitively oriented behavior guidance techniques. For example, teaching patients how to identify and challenge misappraisals of risk or thoughts of disgust may be effective for managing anticipatory anxiety as well as fear reactions in the dental operatory.[33,40,111,115] Given their social development, and compared with younger patients, adolescents may be especially sensitive to embarrassment, which can be a key factor in dental care–related fear and anxiety.[111,116] In using cognitively oriented behavior guidance techniques, and in communicating with adolescents generally, it thus may be particularly useful to attend to potential embarrassment and/or communicate in a nonjudgmental way, carefully considering word choice so as to not provoke embarrassment.

For patients with more significant dental care–related fear and anxiety, and even phobia, exposure-based behavior guidance techniques may be necessary to manage and cure fears and anxieties. Through a mechanism known as extinction learning, repeated exposure to feared stimuli desensitizes patients such that they come to no longer have a fear reaction to the stimuli.[117] The most common exposure-based behavior guidance technique used for dental applications is systematic desensitization, which has been shown to be effective across a range of fears/phobias, including those related to dental stimuli.[117–119] Briefly, patients identify a hierarchy of feared stimuli and are systematically and gradually supported in experiencing those stimuli (moving up the hierarchy) until they habituate and no longer experience a fear response. There is minimal research addressing systematic desensitization for dental care–related fear, anxiety, and phobia among adolescent patients, specifically; however, it is such a robust treatment of fear and anxiety for pediatric and adult populations that it would be considered best practice. The AAPD and numerous experts have offered guidance on the use of systematic desensitization in working with dental patients.[4,32,37,79,107] Moreover, computer-assisted, virtual reality, and single-session approaches to facilitating desensitization have been reported.[120–122]

For dental providers interested in learning more about the behavior guidance techniques discussed earlier, and others, there are numerous meta-analyses, reviews, and books on the topic.[32,37,79,107,123–127] Note that, especially for very fearful or anxious patients, advanced cognitively oriented behavior guidance techniques and systematic desensitization most appropriately may be facilitated by a mental health care provider, in partnership with the dental provider if possible. It is also worth noting that pediatric dental care–related fear and anxiety have been acknowledged as understudied problems.[33] If fear and anxiety are understudied in youth, they are particularly understudied in adolescents. Much more research on the cause, assessment, and management of adolescent dental care–related fear and anxiety is warranted.

INVOLVING A BEHAVIORAL HEALTH PROFESSIONAL

Depending on the severity and impact of dental care–related fear and anxiety experienced by a patient, dental providers may consider referring the patient to a behavioral health professional for adjunctive management. In many cases, behavioral health professionals use the same approaches to assessment and the same behavior guidance techniques described here; however, they often have deeper expertise in and more time to perform such interventions, and **Fig. 1** shows the typical approach.

Patients may be referred to a psychiatrist, a psychologist, a licensed social worker, or a mental health counselor depending on their particular needs and provider availability. There are pediatric specialists working in each of these professions, and some may have particular expertise in working with adolescent patients. Dental professionals are encouraged to become familiar with the types of behavioral health care providers working in their area and to collaborate with behavioral health care providers when shared patients are being treated for dental care–related fear, anxiety, or phobia.

CONSIDERATIONS FOR ADOLESCENTS WITH SPECIAL HEALTH CARE NEEDS

An association between significant medical conditions and dental fear and anxiety in adolescents has not been found.[55] However, specific diseases may have different

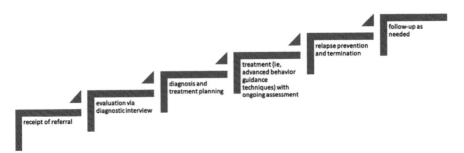

Fig. 1. Typical approach by a behavioral health professional.

impacts. For example, dental fear in patients with cleft lip and/or palate has been well studied, and these patients report higher levels of moderate dental fear compared with general population reports in younger children and in adolescents.[128,129] This fear is likely caused by repeated invasive surgical procedures. Sensitivity in the perioral areas also results in the potential for increased discomfort and pain. Previous medical interventions likely have some impact on dental anxiety, even if individuals do not consciously recognize the association. An anxiety survey of a group of chronically ill adolescents found anxiety levels were significantly higher if the interview was conducted in a medical/dental clinic setting versus a neutral setting (eg, fast food restaurant). Interview location only resulted in a small increase in anxiety for healthy children.[68] Dentists should not underestimate the emotions triggered by medical environments.

Although most adolescents do not require a parent in the operatory, adolescents with developmental special health care needs may benefit from this extra support for reassurance and to enhance communication. A thorough interview to assess cognitive status, medical diagnoses, and social status should be performed. It is important to ask about adolescents' strengths, not just their disabilities.[130] Further, it is important to inquire about sensory sensitivities at the initial interview, and interventions such as dimmed lighting, rhythmic music, and slow-moving visuals can provide a more pleasing environment.[131] Every adolescent is a unique individual and communication should use person-first language. For example, the phrase "a Downs child" could be rephrased as "a child with Down syndrome" to ensure the emphasis is on the person, not the disease.[132]

In recent decades, the right of individuals with special health care needs to make decisions has been emphasized.[130] Adolescents with significant medical conditions without intellectual disability often show a maturity beyond that of their peers. They are often a topic of conversation and may feel objectified in medical and dental settings. Decision-making conversations should be directed toward the patient to establish a therapeutic alliance, and parents should be perceived as supporters in this relationship.

For patients with intellectual disability, communication should be delivered at the appropriate developmental level for the patient, and this may not correlate to chronologic age. Although communication may need to be simplified for comprehension, these adolescents deserve communication directed at them as the patient, and especially communication that shows respect and avoids infantilizing. Use of short, direct communication with single-step instructions is most effective in this group.[130]

Although special health care needs vary dramatically from physical, medical, sensory, or behavioral impairments, there are shared themes. Physical impairments may be compensated for by allowing patients to remain in their wheelchairs, where they typically feel most secure.[130] If a patient needs to be transferred to a dental chair for treatment, the rationale for this need is important, asking for the most comfortable method of transfer, and then special cushioning for support should be used.[130]

For patients with intellectual developmental disorders, behavior guidance techniques have been recognized as patient support techniques to emphasize that person-centered focus should be the basis for these decisions.[133] The techniques that have been most commonly studied are demonstration of behavior, gradual exposure to dental procedures, material reward, and social reward.[133] Many of the typical behavioral guidance techniques for children work well in this group and use should be applied after consideration of cognitive development and potential barriers to implementation.[4]

IMPACT OF CORONAVIRUS DISEASE 2019 PANDEMIC

The impact of the coronavirus disease 2019 (COVID-19) pandemic on the behavior of adolescents in the dental office is still unknown, but it is reasonable to anticipate negative consequences. The unique nature of the lockdown had favorable elements such as increased time with family members, focus on altruism, and freedom from the judgment of their peers. However, the long-term effects of stress and isolation likely outweigh these advantages. Adolescents depend heavily on their peer groups for social interaction, support, and coping, and when this was abruptly withdrawn, the results have been increased anxiety, irritability, and inattention.[134] During the pandemic, mental health challenges worsened with increased substance use and suicidal ideation.[135] Adolescence is a period of vulnerability for the onset of mental illness, with suicide being the third leading cause of morbidity in this age group.[136] During the pandemic, mental health–related emergency department visits for adolescents aged 12 to 17 years increased 31% compared with the previous year.[137]

Vulnerable adolescents may have been disproportionally affected by lack of electronic resources for education and communication and may have been subjected to environments where domestic violence was present.[134] Individuals living in these high-stress environments are at higher risk of developing psychiatric disorders.[134] Likewise, adolescents with special health care needs were also likely disproportionally affected because of an interruption in their ongoing therapies, financial concerns, and fear of contracting COVID-19, although some adolescents viewed the increased time with family members favorably.[138]

As clinicians welcome adolescents back into their offices, it is reasonable to ask parents and the adolescents whether they are aware of any changes in behavior as a result of the pandemic. Adolescents, especially those prone to anxiety, may have unexpressed fears of risk of infection. Asking whether they feel comfortable or have any questions about the safety in the dental office could prompt questions they may otherwise be hesitant to ask. When establishing rapport with patients, remember that typical milestones have been disrupted. If they had challenges with online learning, adolescents may not have been promoted to their typical grades. Rites of passage, such as graduation ceremonies, the prom, and sports, have been canceled. To avoid dwelling on these disappointments, ask about positive developments or what they are most excited about in the future. Dental disease may have progressed because of delayed treatment, and adolescents should be reassured that this was not their fault and that, through a therapeutic alliance, they can still have optimal oral health.

SUMMARY

Adolescence is a period of challenge and potential. Dentists must balance respecting the independence of these emerging adults with supporting them through fears and anxieties that may carry over from childhood or may be emerging during this period of vulnerability. Formal assessment of fear and anxiety should be performed to direct interventions. Communication and the establishment of rapport are critical to the dentist-patient therapeutic alliance in this age group. Other effective techniques take advantage of advancing cognitive-behavioral and other coping skills, such as distraction, breathing exercises, and systematic desensitization.

CLINICS CARE POINTS

- One in 10 adolescents has dental fear or anxiety that may interfere with care seeking.
- Communication techniques that promote active listening and selective information sharing, and instill a sense of control, work well in this age group.
- For patients with severe dental fear or phobia, the dentist should work with a behavioral health provider to prevent avoidance behavior.

REFERENCES

1. Selwitz RH, Ismail AI, Pitts NB. Dental caries. Lancet 2007;369:51–9.
2. Wells MH, McCarthy BA, Tseng C, et al. Usage of behavior guidance techniques differs by provider and practice characteristics. Pediatr Dent 2018;40:201–8.
3. Townsend JA, Wells MH. Behavior guidance of the pediatric dental patient. In: Nowak AJ, Christensen JR, Mabry TR, et al, editors. Pediatric dentistry. 6th edition. Philadelphia: Elsevier; 2019. p. 352–70.
4. American Academy of Pediatric Dentistry. Behavior guidance for the pediatric dental patient. The reference manual of pediatric dentistry. Chicago, IL: American Academy of Pediatric Dentistry; 2020. p. 292–310.
5. Wilson S, Cody WE. An analysis of behavior management papers published in the pediatric dental literature. Pediatr Dent 2005;27:331–8.
6. Mejare IA, Klingberg G, Mowafi FK, et al. A systematic map of systematic reviews in pediatric dentistry–what do we really know? PLoS One 2015;10: e0117537.
7. Thomson WM, Poulton RG, Kruger E, et al. Changes in self-reported dental anxiety in New Zealand adolescents from ages 15 to 18 years. J Dent Res 1997;76: 1287–91.
8. Alderman EM, Breuner CC, American Academy of Pediatrics Committee on Adolescence. Unique needs of the adolescent. Pediatrics 2019;144:e20193150.
9. Giedd JN. Structural magnetic resonance imaging of the adolescent brain. Ann N Y Acad Sci 2004;1021:77–85.
10. Steinberg L. Cognitive and affective development in adolescence. Trends Cogn Sci 2005;9:69–74.
11. Steinberg L, Morris AS. Adolescent development. Annu Rev Psychol 2001;52: 83–110.
12. Giedd JN. The teen brain: insights from neuroimaging. J Adolesc Health 2008; 42:335–43.

13. Hughes K, Bellis MA, Hardcastle KA, et al. The effect of multiple adverse child-hood experiences on health: a systematic review and meta-analysis. Lancet Public Health 2017;2:e356–66.

14. Smetana JG, Campione-Barr N, Metzger A. Adolescent development in inter-personal and societal contexts. Annu Rev Psychol 2006;57:255–84.

15. Collins WA, Laursen B. Parent-adolescent relationships and influences. In: Lerner RM, Steinberg L, editors. Handbook of adolescent psychology. Hobo-ken, NJ: Wiley; 2004. p. 331–61.

16. Youniss J, Smollar JM. Adolescents' relations with mothers, fathers, and friends. Chicago: Chicago Press; 1985. p. 1–14.

17. Adams R, Laursen B. The organization and dynamics of adolescent conflict with parents and friends. J Marriage Fam 2001;63:97–110.

18. Larson R, Richards MH. Daily companionship in late childhood and early adolescence: changing developmental contexts. Child Dev 1991;62:284–300.

19. Furman W, Buhrmester D. Age and sex differences in perceptions of networks of personal relationships. Child Dev 1992;63:103–15.

20. Choudhury S, Blakemore SJ, Charman T. Social cognitive development during adolescence. Soc Cogn Affect Neurosci 2006;1:165–74.

21. Coleman JC. The self and identity. In: The nature of adolescence. East Sussex, UK: Routledge; 2011. p. 57–78.

22. Harter S, Monsour A. Development analysis of conflict caused by opposing at-tributes in the adolescent self-portrait. Dev Psychol 1992;28:251–60.

23. Burdette AM, Needham BL, Taylor MG, et al. Health lifestyles in adolescence and self-rated health into adulthood. J Health Soc Behav 2017;58:520–36.

24. Hargreaves DS, Elliott MN, Viner RM, et al. Unmet health care need in US ado-lescents and adult health outcomes. Pediatrics 2015;136:513–20.

25. Park MJ, Adams SH, Irwin CE. Health care services and the transition to young adulthood: challenges and opportunities. Acad Pediatr 2011;11:115–22.

26. Umberson D, Crosnoe R, Reczek C. Social relationships and health behavior across the life course. Annu Rev Soc 2010;36:139–57.

27. National Institute of Dental and Craniofacial Research. Interdisciplinary ap-proaches to promote adolescents' oral health and reduce disparities. 2020. Available at: https://www.nidcr.nih.gov/grants-funding/funding-priorities/future-research-initiatives/interdisciplinary-approaches-promote-adolescents-oral-health-reduce-disparities. Accessed February 19, 2021.

28. Armfield J. How do we measure dental fear and what are we measuring any-way? Oral Health Prev Dent 2010;8:107–15.

29. Asl AN, Shokravi M, Jamali Z, et al. Barriers and drawbacks of the assessment of dental fear, dental anxiety, and dental phobia in children: a critical literature review. J Clin Pediatr Dent 2017;41:399–423.

30. McNeil DW, Arias MC, Randall CL. Anxiety versus fear. In: Wenzel AE, Frideman-Wheeler D, Flannery-Schroeder E, editors. Encyclopedia of abnormal and clin-ical psychology. Thousand Oaks, CA: Sage; 2017. p. 279–80.

31. Craske MG. Origins of phobias and anxiety disorders: why more women than men? Oxford: Elsevier Ltd; 2003.

32. McNeil DW, Randall CL. Dental fear and anxiety associated with oral health care: conceptual and clinical issues. In: Mostofsky D, Fortune A, editors. Behav-ioral dentistry. Ames, IA: John Wiley & Sons, Inc; 2014. p. 165–92.

33. Seligman LD, Hovey JD, Chacon K, et al. Dental anxiety: an understudied prob-lem in youth. Clin Psychol Rev 2017;55:25–40.

34. Carter AE, Carter G, Boschen M, et al. Pathways of fear and anxiety in dentistry: a review. World J Clin Cases 2014;2:642–53.

35. Klingberg G, Arnrup K. Dental fear and behavior management problems. In: Koch G, Poulsen S, Espelid I, et al, editors. Pediatric dentistry: a clinical approach. West Sussex, UK: John Wiley & Sons, Ltd; 2017. p. 55–65.

36. Klingberg G, Broberg AG. Dental fear/anxiety and dental behaviour management problems in children and adolescents: a review of prevalence and concomitant psychological factors. Pediatr Dent 2007;17:391–406.

37. Milgrom P, Weinstein P, Heaton LJ. Treating fearful dental patients: a patient management handbook. Seattle, WA: Dental Behavioral Resources; 2009.

38. Berggren U, Carlsson SG, Hagglin C, et al. Assessment of patients with direct conditioned and indirect cognitive reported origin of dental fear. Eur J Oral Sci 1997;105:213–20.

39. Davey GC. Dental phobias and anxieties: evidence for conditioning processes in the acquisition and modulation of a learned fear. Behav Res Ther 1989; 27:51–8.

40. de Jongh A, Muris P, ter Horst G, et al. Acquisition and maintenance of dental anxiety: the role of conditioning experiences and cognitive factors. Behav Res Ther 1995;33:205–10.

41. Liddell A, Locker D. Changes in levels of dental anxiety as a function of dental experience. Behav Modif 2000;24:57–68.

42. Locker D, Liddell A, Dempster L, et al. Age of onset of dental anxiety. J Dent Res 1999;78:790–6.

43. Mares J, Hesova M, Skalska H, et al. Children pain during dental treatment. Acta Med 1997;40:103–8.

44. Melamed BG, Williamson DJ. Programs for the treatment of dental disorders: dental anxiety and temporomandibular disorders. In: Sweet J, Rozensky R, Tovian S, editors. Handbook of psychology in medical settings. New York: Plenum Press; 1991. p. 539–65.

45. Abrahamsson KH, Ohrn K, Hakeberg M. Dental beliefs: factor structure of the revised dental beliefs survey in a group of regular dental patients. Eur J Oral Sci 2009;117:720–7.

46. Chapman HR, Kirby-Turner NC. The treatment of dental fear in children and adolescents – a cognitive-behavioral approach to the development of coping skills and their clinical application. In: Gower PL, editor. New research on the psychology of fear. Hauppauge, NY: Nova Science Publishers; 2005. p. 105–40.

47. de Jongh A, Murs P, ter Horst G, et al. Cognitive correlates of dental anxiety. J Dent Res 1994;73:561–6.

48. Doerr PA, Lang WP, Nyquist LV, et al. Factors associated with dental anxiety. J Am Dent Assoc 1998;129:1111–9.

49. Armfield J. Towards a better understanding of dental anxiety and fear: cognition vs. experiences. Eur J Oral Sci 2010;118:259–64.

50. Milgrom P, Vignehsa H, Weinstein P. Adolescent dental fear and control: prevalence and theoretical implications. Behav Res Ther 1992;30:367–73.

51. Arnup K, Broberg AG, Berggren U, et al. Lack of cooperation in pediatric dentistry – the role of child personality characteristics. Pediatr Dent 2002;24: 119–28.

52. Cianetti S, Lombardo G, Lupatelli E, et al. Dental fear/anxiety among children and adolescents. A systematic review. Eur J Paediatr Dent 2017;18:121–30.

53. Baier K, Milgrom P, Russell S, et al. Children's fear and behavior in private pediatric dentistry practices. Pediatr Dent 2004;26:316–21.

54. Alshoraim MA, El-Housseiny AA, Farsi NM, et al. Effects of child characteristics and dental history on dental fear: cross-sectional study. BMC Oral Health 2018; 18:33.
55. Alvesalo I, Murtomaa H, Milgrom P, et al. The dental fear survey schedule: a study with finish children. Int J Paediatr Dent 1993;3:193–8.
56. Bedi R, Sutcliffe P, Donnan PT, et al. The prevalence of dental anxiety in a group of 13-14-year-old Scottish children. Int J Paediatr Dent 1992;2:17–24.
57. Bergius M, Berggren U, Bogdanov O, et al. Dental anxiety among adolescents in St. Petersburg Russia. Eur J Oral Sci 1997;105:117–22.
58. Chellappah NK, Bignesha H, Milgrom P, et al. Prevalence of dental anxiety and fear in children in Singapore. Community Dent Oral Epidemiol 1990;18:269–71.
59. Lara A, Crego A, Romero-Maroto M. Emotional contagion of dental fear to children: the fathers' mediating role in parental transfer of fear. Int J Paediatr Dent 2012;22:324–30.
60. Lin Y, Yen Y, Chen H, et al. Child dental fear in low-income and non-low-income families: a school-based survey study. J Dent Sci 2014;9:165–71.
61. Luoto A, Tolvanen M, Pojola V, et al. A longitudinal study of changes and associations in dental fear in parent/adolescent dyads. Int J Paediatr Dent 2017; 27(6):506–13.
62. Nakai Y, Hirakawa T, Milgrom P, et al. The children's fear survey schedule-dental subscale in Japan. Community Dent Oral Epidemiol 2005;33:196–204.
63. Peretz B, Efrat J. Dental anxiety among young adolescent patients in Israel. Int J Paediatr Dent 2000;10:126–32.
64. Taani DQ, El-Qaderi SS, Abu Alhaija ESJ. Dental anxiety in children and its relationship to dental caries and gingival condition. Int J Dent Hyg 2005;3:83–7.
65. Majstorovic M, Morse DE, Do D, et al. Indicators of dental anxiety in children just prior to treatment. J Clin Pediatri Dent 2014;39:12–7.
66. Dogan MC, Seydaoglu G, Uguz S, et al. The effect of age, gender and socioeconomic factors on perceived dental anxiety determined by a modified scale in children. Oral Health Prev Dent 2006;4:235–41.
67. Holst A, Crossner CG. Direct ratings of acceptance of dental treatment in Swedish children. Community Dent Oral Epidemiol 1987;15:258–63.
68. Walton JW, Johnson SB, Algina J. Mother and child perceptions of child anxiety: effects of race, health status, and stress. J Pediatr Psych 1999;24:29–39.
69. Karibe H, Kato Y, Shimazu K, et al. Gender differences in adolescents' perceptions toward dentists using the Japanese version of the dental beliefs survey: a cross-sectional survey. BMC Oral Health 2019;19:144.
70. Skaret E, Raadal M, Berg E, et al. Dental anxiety and dental avoidance among 12 to 18 year olds in Norway. Eur J Oral Sci 1999;107:422–8.
71. Murray P, Liddell A, Donohue J. A longitudinal study of the contribution of dental experience to dental anxiety in children between 9 and 12 years of age. J Behav Med 1989;12:309–20.
72. McNeil DW, Randall CL, Cohen LL, et al. Transmission of dental fear from parent to adolescent in an Appalachian sample in the USA. Int J Paediatr Dent 2019;29: 720–7.
73. Vika M, Skaret E, Raadal M, et al. Fear of blood, injury, and injections, and its relationship to dental anxiety and probability of avoiding dental treatment among 18-year-olds in Norway. Int J Paediatr Dent 2008;18:163–9.
74. Alwin N, Murray JJ, Britton PG. An assessment of dental anxiety in children. Br Dent J 1991;171:201–7.

75. Locker D, Poulton R, Thomson WM. Psychological disorders and dental anxiety in a young adult population. Community Dent Oral Epidemiol 2001;29:456–63.
76. Creswell C, Waite P, Cooper PJ. Assessment and management of anxiety disorders in children and adolescents. Arch Dis Child 2014;99:674–8.
77. Sharif MO. Dental anxiety: detection and management. J Appl Oral Sci 2010; 18:i.
78. Alshammasi H, Buchanan H, Ashley P. Dentists' use of validated child dental anxiety measures in clinical practice: a mixed methods study. Int J Paediatr Dent 2018;28:62–71.
79. Armfield JM, Heaton LJ. Management of fear and anxiety in the dental clinic: a review. Aust Dent J 2013;58:390–407.
80. Dailey YM, Humphris GM, Lennon MA. The use of dental anxiety questionnaires: a survey of a group of UK dental practitioners. Br Dent J 2001;190:450–3.
81. Heaton LJ, Carlson CR, Smith TA, et al. Predicting anxiety during dental treatment using patients' self-reports: less is more. J Am Dent Assoc 2007;138: 188–95.
82. Holmes RD, Girdler NM. A study to assess the validity of clinical judgement in determining paediatric dental anxiety and related outcomes of management. Int J Paediatr Dent 2005;15:169–76.
83. Hoglund M, Bagesund M, Shahnavaz S, et al. Evaluation of the ability of dental clinicians to rate dental anxiety. Eur J Oral Sci 2019;127:455–61.
84. Porritt J, Buchanan H, Hall M, et al. Assessing children's dental anxiety: a systematic review of current measures. Community Dent Oral Epidemiol 2013;41: 130–42.
85. Yon MJY, Chen KJ, Gao SS, et al. An introduction to assessing dental fear and anxiety in children. Healthcare 2020;8:86.
86. Conijn JM, Smits N, Hartman EE. Determining at what age children provide sound self-reports: an illustration of the validity-index approach. Assessment 2020;27:1604–18.
87. Howard KE, Freeman R. Reliability and validity of a faces version of the Modified Child Dental Anxiety Scale. Int J Paediatr Dent 2007;17:281–8.
88. Mellor D, Moore KA. The use of Likert scales with children. J Pediatr Psychol 2014;39:369–79.
89. Muris P, Ollendick TH. The assessment of contemporary fears in adolescents using a modified version of the Fear Survey Schedule for Children-Revised. J Anxiety Disord 2002;16:567–84.
90. Wong HM, Humphris GM, Lee GTR. Preliminary validation and reliability of the modified child dental anxiety scale. Psychol Rep 1998;83:1179–86.
91. Coombes L, Bristowe K, Ellis-Smith C, et al. Enhancing validity, reliability and participation in self-reported health outcome measurement for children and young people: a systematic review of recall period, response scale format, and administration modality. Qual Life Res 2021. https://doi.org/10.1007/s11136-021-02814-4.
92. Humphris GM, Morrison T, Lindsay SJ. The Modified Dental Anxiety Scale: validation and United Kingdom norms. Community Dent Health 1995;12:143–50.
93. Honkala S, Al-Yahya H, Honkala E, et al. Validating a measure of the prevalence of dental anxiety as applied to Kuwaiti adolescents. Community Dent Health 2014;31:251–6.
94. Newton JT, Buck DJ. Anxiety and pain measures in dentistry: a guide to their quality and application. J Am Dent Assoc 2000;131:1449–57.

95. Wong HM, Peng SM, Perfecto A, et al. Dental anxiety and caries experience from late childhood through adolescence to early adulthood. Community Dent Oral Epidemiol 2020;48:513–21.

96. Kleinknecht R, Klepac R, Alexander LD. Origins and characteristics of fear of dentistry. J Dent Res 1973;86:842–8.

97. Kleinknecht R, Thorndike RM, McGlynn FD, et al. Factor analysis of the dental fear survey with cross-validation. J Am Dent Assoc 1984;108:59–61.

98. Smith T, Moore RA. Repression of dental anxiety. J Dent Res 1995;74:144.

99. Gauthier JG, Ricard S, Morin BA, et al. Adolescents' fear of dental treatment: development and evaluation of a cognitive inventory. J Can Dent Assoc 1991; 57:658–62.

100. Buchanan H, Niven N. Validation of a Facial Image Scale to assess child dental anxiety. Int J Paediatr Dent 2002;12(1):47–52.

101. Cuthbert MI, Melamed BG. A screening device: children at risk for dental fear and management problems. J Dent Child 1982;49:432–6.

102. Kent G, Croucher R. Achieving oral health: the social context of dental care. Oxford: Butterworth Heinemann; 1998.

103. Alvarez E, Puliafica A, Leonte KG, et al. Psychotherapy for anxiety disorders in children and adolescents. Up to Date; 2021. Available at: https://www.uptodate.com/contents/psychotherapy-for-anxiety-disorders-in-children-and-adolescents. Accessed May 5, 2021.

104. Neverlein PO, Backer Johnsen T. Optimism-pessimism dimension and dental anxiety in children aged 10-12 years. Community Dent Oral Epidemiol 1991; 19:342–6.

105. Hamzah HS, Gao X, Yung Yiu CK, et al. Managing dental fear and anxiety in pediatric patients: a qualitative study from the public's perspective. Pediatr Dent 2014;36:29–33.

106. Nash DA. Engaging children's cooperation in the dental environment through effective communication. Pediatr Dent 2006;28:455–9.

107. Weiner AA. The fearful dental patient: a guide to understanding and managing. Ames: Wiley-Blackwell; 2011.

108. Logan HL, Baron RS, Keeley K, et al. Desired control and felt control as mediators of stress in a dental setting. Health Psychol 1991;10:532–9.

109. Lidell A, Locker D. Gender and age differences in attitudes to dental pain and dental control. Comm Dent Oral Epidemol 1997;25:314–8.

110. Rollnick S, Butler CC, Kinnersley, et al. Motivational interviewing. BMJ 2010;340: c1900.

111. Berggren U, Hakeberg M, Carlsson SG. Relaxation vs. cognitively oriented therapies for dental fear. J Dent Res 2000;79(9):1645–51.

112. Fried R. The role of respiration in stress and stress control: toward a theory of stress as a hypoxic phenomenon. In: Lehrer PM, Woolfolk RL, editors. Principles and practices of stress management. New York: Guilford; 1993. p. 301–30.

113. Liu Y, Gu Z, Wang Y, et al. Effect of audiovisual distraction on the management of dental anxiety in children: a systematic review. Int J Paediatr Dent 2019;29: 14–21.

114. Prado IM, Carcavalli L, Abreu LG, et al. Use of distraction techniques for the management of anxiety and fear in paediatric dental practice: a systematic review of randomized controlled trials. Int J Paediatr Dent 2019;29:650–68.

115. Armfield JM, Slade GD, Spencer AJ. Cognitive vulnerability and dental fear. BMC Oral Health 2008;8:2.

116. Moore R, Brodsgaard I, Rosenberg N. The contribution of embarrassment to phobic dental anxiety: a qualitative research study. BMC Psychiatry 2004;4:10.

117. Craske MG, Hermans D, Vansteenwegen D. Fear and learning: from basic processes to clinical implications. Washington, DC: American Psychological on; 2006. p. 217–34.

118. Choy Y, Fyer AJ, Lipsitz JD. Treatment of specific phobia in adults. Clin Psychol Rev 2007;27(3):266–86.

119. Hakeberg M, Berggren U, Carlsson SG. A 10-year follow-up of patients treated for dental fear. Scand J Dent Res 1990;98:53–9.

120. Coldwell SE, Getz T, Milgrom P, et al. CARL: a LabVIEW 3 computer program for conducting exposure therapy for the treatment of dental injection fear. J Anxiety Disord 2007;21:871–87.

121. Ost LG. One-session treatment for specific phobias. Behav Res Ther 1989; 27:1–7.

122. Raghav K, van Wijk AJ, Abdullah F, et al. Efficacy of virtual reality exposure therapy for treatment of dental phobia: a randomized control trial. BMC Oral Health 2016;16:25.

123. Appukuttan DP. Strategies to manage patients with dental anxiety and dental phobia: literature review. Clin Cosmet Investig Dent 2016;10:35–50.

124. Gordon D, Heimberg RG, Tellez M, et al. A critical review of approaches to the treatment of dental anxiety in adults. J Anxiety Disord 2013;27:365–78.

125. Kvale G, Berggren U, Milgrom P. Dental fear in adults: a meta-analysis of behavioral interventions. Community Dent Oral Epidemiol 2004;32:250–64.

126. Ost LG, Skaret E. Cognitive behavioral therapy for dental phobia and anxiety. West Sussex, UK: John Wiley & Sons, Ltd; 2013.

127. Wide Boman U, Carlsson V, Westin M, et al. Psychological treatment of dental anxiety among adults: a systematic review. Eur J Oral Sci 2013;121:225–34.

128. Vogels W, Aartman I, Veerkamp J. Dental fear in children with a cleft lip and/or cleft palate. Cleft Palate Craniofac J 2011;48:6.

129. Mirjami C, Saujanya K, Virpi H, et al. Dental fear among adolescents with cleft. Int J Paediatr Dent 2012. https://doi.org/10.1111/ipd.12782.

130. Klingberg G. Children with disabilities. In: Wright GZ, Kupietzky A, editors. Behavior management in dentistry for children. 2nd edition. Ames: Wiley Blackwell; 2014. p. 93–105.

131. Shapiro M, Sgan-Cohen HD, Parush S, et al. Influence of adapted environment on the anxiety of medically treated children with developmental disability. J Pediatr 2009;154:546–50.

132. Webb JR. Overview of disability. In: Nelson TM, Webb JR, editors. Dental care for children with special needs: a clinical guide. Cham, Switzerland: Springer; 2019. p. 1–26.

133. Phadraig CMG, Asimakopolou K, Daly B, et al. Nonpharmacological techniques to support patients with intellectual developmental disorders to receive dental treatment: a systematic review of behavior change techniques. Spec Care Dentist 2020;40:10–25.

134. de Figueiredo CS, Sandre PC, Portugal LCL, et al. COVID-19 pandemic impact on children and adolescents' mental health: Biological, environmental, and social factors. Prog Neuropsychopharmacol Biol Psychiatry 2021;106:110171.

135. Czeisler MÉ, Lane RI, Petrosky E, et al. Mental health, substance use, and suicidal ideation during the COVID-19 pandemic - United States, June 24-30, 2020. MMWR Morb Mortal Wkly Rep 2020;69:1049–57.

136. Shah K, Mann S, Singh R, et al. Impact of COVID-19 on the mental health of children and adolescents. Cureus 2020;12:e10051.

137. Leeb RT, Bitsko RH, Radhakrishnan L, et al. Mental health-related emergency department visits among children aged <18 years during the COVID-19 pandemic - United States, January 1-October 17, 2020. MMWR Morb Mortal Wkly Rep 2020;69:1675–80.

138. Faccioli S, Lombardi F, Bellini P. How did Italian adolescents with disability and parents deal with the COVID-19 emergency? Int J Environ Res Public Health 2021;18(4):1687.

Sedation and Anesthesia for the Adolescent Dental Patient

Matthew Cooke, DDS, MD, MPH[a,b,*], Thomas Tanbonliong, DDS[c]

KEYWORDS

- Sedation • Anxiolysis • Anesthesia • Adolescent dental patient
- Prescribing considerations • Rescue • Obesity
- Attention-deficit/hyperactivity disorder

KEY POINTS

- This article aims to help clinicians with indications and contraindications for sedation and anesthesia of adolescent dental patients.
- The article presents the spectrum of sedation and anesthesia in adolescent dentistry.
- A review of basic pharmacology of sedation/anesthesia agents and the concept of rescue is presented.
- Techniques require individualization. Challenges associated with perioperative management of adolescent dental patients as they relate to risk and benefit should be considered.

INTRODUCTION

Dentists who provide sedation or anesthesia to adolescent dental patients are urged to have current knowledge of pharmacology. They must recognize indications and contraindications to the delivery of sedation and anesthesia medications, including epinephrine-containing local
anesthetics. Management of pain, anxiety, and behavior should be the goals of sedation/anesthesia. All decisions must be made considering risk versus benefit.

Dentists are obligated to use safe prescribing practices. The goal of this article is to aid the dental provider in managing pain and anxiety and in modifying behavior to safely complete dental procedures in adolescent patients.

[a] Department of Dental Anesthesiology, School of Dental Medicine, University of Pittsburgh, 3501 Terrace Street, Pittsburgh, PA 15261, USA; [b] Department of Pediatric Dentistry, School of Dental Medicine, University of Pittsburgh, 3501 Terrace Street, Pittsburgh, PA 15261, USA; [c] Division of Pediatric Dentistry, Department of Orofacial Sciences, University of California San Francisco, School of Dentistry, Box 0753, 707 Parnassus Avenue, D-1021, San Francisco, CA 94143, USA
* Corresponding author. Departments of Dental Anesthesiology & Pediatric Dentistry, School of Dental Medicine, University of Pittsburgh, 3501 Terrace Street, Pittsburgh, PA 15261.
E-mail address: mrc99@pitt.edu

Dent Clin N Am 65 (2021) 753–773
https://doi.org/10.1016/j.cden.2021.07.004
0011-8532/21/© 2021 Elsevier Inc. All rights reserved.

dental.theclinics.com

DEFINITIONS

There have been many definitions of sedation in dentistry used over the years. Clinical standards for sedation in dentistry parallel the guidelines established by the American Society of Anesthesiology (ASA) for anesthesiologists.[1,2] The American Academy of Pediatric Dentistry (AAPD) and the Academy of Pediatrics (AAP) maintain guidelines for sedation of the pediatric patient, defined as any patient under the age of 21.[3] The American Dental Association (ADA) also has guidelines for the use and teaching of sedation and anesthesia in dentistry.[4–6]

The following definitions for levels of sedation are excerpted from the AAPD, AAP, and ADA guidelines.[3–6]

Minimal Sedation

(Old terminology was "anxiolysis"): A pharmacologic-induced state that retains a patient's ability to respond normally to tactile stimulation and verbal command. Cognitive function and coordination may be impaired; ventilatory and cardiovascular functions are unaffected.

Moderate Sedation

(Old terminology was "conscious sedation" or "sedation/analgesia"): a drug-induced depression of consciousness during which patients respond purposefully to verbal commands (eg, "open your eyes" either alone or accompanied by light tactile stimulation, such as a light tap on the shoulder, not a sternal rub). For older patients, this level of sedation implies an interactive state; for younger patients, age-appropriate behaviors occur and are expected.

Note: "the drug(s) and/or techniques used should carry a margin of safety wide enough to render loss of consciousness unlikely."[7]

Deep Sedation

A drug-induced depression of consciousness during which patients cannot be easily aroused but respond purposefully after repeated verbal or painful stimulation. The ability to independently maintain ventilatory function may be impaired. Patients may require assistance in maintaining a patent airway, and spontaneous ventilation may be inadequate. Cardiovascular function is usually maintained. A state of deep sedation may be accompanied by partial or complete loss of protective reflexes.

General Anesthesia

A drug-induced loss of consciousness during which patients are not arousable, even by painful stimulation. The ability to independently maintain ventilatory function is often impaired. Patients often require assistance in maintaining a patent airway, and positive pressure ventilation may be required because of depressed spontaneous ventilation or drug-induced depression of neuromuscular function. Cardiovascular function may be impaired.

SPECTRUM OF ANESTHESIA AND SEDATION

Arthur Guedel, MD introduced the concept of anesthetic signs and stages. His early work studied diethyl ether for general anesthesia. He observed 4 distinct stages as patients were administered increasing quantities of inhaled ether. The stages represent a continuum or spectrum from which no sedation becomes general anesthesia.[8,9]

In stage 1 or the analgesia phase, consciousness is not lost. Stage 2 is the excitatory phase. Between stages 2 and 3, consciousness is lost. Stage 3 is defined as the surgical anesthesia stage. *Dentists who are not formally trained in deep sedation and general anesthesia should limit their practice to stage 1, the analgesia phase.*

Guedel's classification still has value. It has been modified and adapted for new drugs and techniques. Dentists must understand that as agents are administered, they produce an effect along a *"spectrum of pain and anxiety control."*[7] Dosage and route determine the level of sedation or anesthesia.

Fig. 1 shows the spectrum. At the far left, there is no sedation or anesthesia. To the right, there are levels of conscious sedation up to the vertical bar. The red bar represents loss of consciousness. To the right of the red bar is deep sedation/general anesthesia. The experienced provider may not need a graphic representation to determine level of sedation or anesthesia; however, a classification system is necessary. The dentist must understand where he or she is on the spectrum and its relationship to where they want to be. Success in the minimal-moderate range is dependent on adequate pain control with local anesthesia. Increasing depth of sedation increases risk and requires additional formal training.

Rescue

"Rescue" is an essential concept of safe sedation. Because sedation and anesthesia are a continuum, a provider must be able to recover a patient from unintended entry to a more profound level of central nervous system (CNS) depression.[3,7,10,11] The ASA's guidelines for sedation by "nonanesthesiologists" stress this concept in an effort to reduce morbidity and mortality.[1,2]

Because sedation and general anesthesia are a continuum, it is not always possible to predict how an individual patient will respond. Hence, practitioners intending to produce a given level of sedation should be able to diagnose and manage the physiologic consequences (rescue) for patients whose level of sedation becomes deeper than initially intended.[1,2,4–6]

For all levels of sedation, the qualified dentist must have the training, skills, drugs and equipment to identify and manage such an occurrence until either assistance arrives (emergency medical service) or the patient returns to the intended level of sedation without airway or cardiovascular complications.[1,2,4–6]

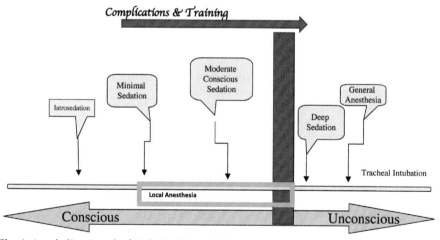

Fig. 1. Levels (Spectrum) of Sedation/Anesthesia.

Sedation without drugs is iatrosedation. Techniques include acupressure, acupuncture, biofeedback, electronic dental anesthesia, and hypnosis.[7] These modalities may be an alternative to traditional sedation/anesthesia for adolescent dental patients. However, for purposes of this article, the authors focus on the use of pharmacotherapy to obtain a desired outcome.

Communication improves outcome. There is no substitute for good verbal and nonverbal communication in adolescent dentistry. The style should be developmentally age-appropriate and nonjudgmental. Good communication alleviates fear and anxiety, allowing treatment to proceed in a "normal" fashion.[7] Traditional behavior management/guidance techniques, such as distraction, tell-show-do, guided imagery, topical anesthesia, and hypnosis, may reduce the need for or depth of pharmacologic sedation.[3,12] *Adolescent dental patients benefit from effective communication.*

PREOPERATIVE EVALUATION

Dental treatment can affect both the physical and the psychological "well-being" of adolescent patients. Before treatment (with or without sedation), patients should have a complete physical examination and psychological assessment to evaluate risk. This assessment allows the provider to determine need.

Medical, dental, and psychological histories guide the dentist in choosing a treatment modality. The evaluation should include a medical history questionnaire, physical examination, and a discussion with the patient, parent, and/or caregiver. For the adolescent patient, extra time and attention should be spent on understanding the reason for their behavior (fear, anxiety, developmental disability). With the information collected, the dentist can establish a physical status classification and determine risk factors. Medical consults can be obtained as needed.[7]

A preoperative consult/evaluation with a physician is not medical clearance. The purpose is to evaluate and make recommendations. Preoperative goals include medical optimization using strategies to reduce risk and improve outcome.[13,14]

PHYSICAL STATUS CLASSIFICATION

The ASA has a physical classification system for estimating medical risk for patients receiving general anesthesia for surgical procedures.[15] The system was adopted in the early 1960s and has remained virtually unchanged. Currently, it is used to evaluate risk associated with procedures regardless of anesthetic technique.[16,17]

The ASA Physical Status Classification System[15]:

Class 1: A healthy patient (no physiologic, physical or psychological abnormalities)

Class 2: A patient with mild systemic disease without limitation of daily activities (ie, controlled asthma; controlled hypertension)

Class 3: A patient with severe systemic disease that limits activity but is not incapacitating (ie, uncontrolled hypertension: uncontrolled diabetes)

Class 4: A patient with incapacitating systemic disease that is a constant threat to life

Class 5: A moribund patient not expected to survive without the operation

Class 6: A brain-dead patient whose organs are being removed for donor purposes

*If the procedure to be performed is an emergency, an "E" is added to the above classification system (eg, ASA PS 2E). In the outpatient medical and dental settings, classes 5 and 6 have been eliminated.[15]

Adolescent patients who are ASA PS class 1 or 2 are appropriate candidates for minimal, moderate, or deep sedation in the dental office.[3] Individual consideration is recommended for patients in ASA PS classes 3 and 4.[3,18] Dentists are encouraged to consult with appropriate subspecialties for patients at increased risk for adverse events because of their underlying conditions. Remember, the ultimate responsibility and liability rest with the dentist who decides to treat or not treat.

SEDATION

Sedation of adolescent patients for the delivery of oral health care uniquely is challenging. A sedation plan should maximize benefit and minimize associated risks for adverse outcomes. Each sedation patient requires individual consideration. Patient extremes in responsiveness and acceptance will vary depending on a host of factors.

Clinical Considerations:
The ideal sedation should

1. Be safe

2. Be easy to administer

3. Have rapid and reliable onset

4. Alleviate pain and anxiety

5. Have minimal undesirable sided effects

6. Be reversible

Once pharmacosedation is planned, the dentist must consider which agents to use and how to administer. The choice will depend on the desired level of sedation. Developmental and chronologic ages are important considerations. Younger patients and severely developmentally disabled patients may require deeper levels of sedation to gain control of their behavior as compared with more cooperative patients.[3]

The following routes are available for delivery of drugs to adolescent patients:

1. Oral/rectal
2. Sublingual
3. Topical
4. Intranasal
5. Inhalational
6. Subcutaneous
7. Intramuscular (IM)
8. Intravenous (IV)
9. Interarterial
10. Intrathecal (in spinal fluid)
11. Transdermal (through epidermis)

Techniques (oral, rectal, sublingual) that administer agents that are absorbed through the gastrointestinal (GI) tract or oral mucosa are termed enteral sedation. Parenteral techniques (IM, IV, intranasal, submucosal, subcutaneous, intraosseous) bypass the gastrointestinal tract and enter directly into the systemic circulation.[4–6] Oral (mostly) and rectal routes are subject to the enterohepatic circulation and first-pass effect before the drug is released to the systemic circulation. This significantly reduces the amount that is bioavailable and should be considered when choosing an agent and dose.[7]

The most popular route used for dental sedation is the oral route. Advantages over the parenteral routes include acceptance by patients, low cost, ease of administration, decreased incidence of adverse reactions, and no equipment needed for delivery.[7] However, oral sedation does have some significant disadvantages, such as reliance on patient compliance, a prolonged latent period, erratic and incomplete absorption from the GI tract, inability to titrate, inability to lighten or deepen sedation as needed, and a prolonged duration of action. *With oral sedation, "stacking" or adding additional agents after the initial dose is discouraged.*

Drugs administered topically are readily absorbed from nonkeratinized tissue. Topical applications in dentistry are usually local anesthetics. They are highly effective at relieving pain associated with intraoral injections.[19]

Intranasal administration has become increasingly popular in pediatric dentistry. It is easily administered to resistant, uncooperative, or precooperative patients.[7,20–22] Although there is brief discomfort with administration, direct absorption into the systemic circulation makes the drug rapidly bioavailable. Compared with oral sedation, there is reduced time to onset and total time spent in the office. Midazolam, a water-soluble benzodiazepine, is a commonly used drug via this route.[7,20–23] The mucosal atomization device is the preferred method for administration.

Inhalational administration occurs when gaseous agents pass from the respiratory apparatus (nose/mouth, trachea, and lungs) into the cardiovascular system. There are a variety of agents available for inhalational sedation and anesthesia. In dentistry, nitrous oxide/oxygen (N_2O/O_2) sedation is the main drug used for inhalation sedation.[7,24] It is easily titrated to effect, with minimal side effects or complications. A disadvantage of nitrous oxide is that it is not a potent anesthetic, so there may be failure. Also, a delivery system is required with a fail-safe and scavenging system. The equipment must be calibrated annually, and there needs to be adequate office ventilation to prevent chronic exposure to those administering the sedation. Other more potent inhalation agents include sevoflurane, isoflurane, and desflurane. They are used in the maintenance of general anesthesia.[7] Sevoflurane is also indicated for mask induction of general anesthesia.

Subcutaneous injection is administration of a drug beneath the skin into the subcutaneous tissue. Rate of absorption is directly proportional to the vasculature in the area of injection. Slow rates of absorption limit its usefulness in dentistry.

The IM route administers the drug directly into the muscle. This parenteral technique allows for quick onset with rapid maximal clinical effect. The disadvantages include prolonged deep sedation, injury to tissues at the site of injection, and overdose. IM administration is often unpredictable, and there is no mechanism for titration to effect. Ketamine, a dissociative anesthetic, is the most commonly used drug via the IM route and is often used for sedation and induction of the uncooperative patient.[25]

Intravascular drug administration represents the most effective, predictable method of delivery for adequate sedation of most patients.[7] Advantages include rapid onset with short duration of latency and a shortened recovery period. However, complications at the site of venipuncture and risk for overdose are disadvantages. Many drugs given intravenously do not have reversal agents; therefore, the dentist must be prepared to manage deeper sedation and other complications, such as allergic reactions, which may not be seen with other less effective modes of delivery.[7]

A variety of drugs are available for sedation and anesthesia of the adolescent patient. These drugs primarily include inhalation sedation/anesthesia, benzodiazepines, sedative hypnotics, antihistamines, alpha agonists, and analgesics. **Table 1** lists available drugs for sedation.

Table 1	
Agents available for adolescent dental sedation/anesthesia	

Alpha agonists
  Clonidine
  Dexmedetomidine
	Anticholinergics
	  Atropine
	  Scopolamine
	  Glycopyrrolate

Antihistamines
  Hydroxyzine
  Diphenhydramine
  Promethazine
	Barbiturates
	  Methohexital
	  Sodium thiopental

Benzodiazepines
  Diazepam
  Midazolam
  Lorazepam
  Triazolam
	Dissociative anesthetics
	  Ketamine[a]

Hypnotics
  Chloral hydrate
	Opioid agonists
	  Fentanyl
	  Morphine
	  Meperidine
	  Alfentanil,[a] sufentanil,[a] remifentanil[a]

Nonnarcotic analgesics
  Acetaminophen
  Ketorolac
	Propofol[a]

[a] Not recommended for use in IV moderate sedation without anesthesia training.

The sedation/anesthetic regimen for adolescent dental patients should carry a high therapeutic index with a wide safety margin and a low probability for abuse. It should be modified based on the adolescent's physical, developmental, mental, sensory, behavioral, cognitive, and emotional needs. Selection of the fewest agents paired with the procedural goals results in safe practice.[26–31] Painful procedures require analgesics; diagnostic procedures use sedatives, and anxious patients benefit from benzodiazepines. Combinations of different classes of medications are often used. However, when 3 or more agents are administered simultaneously, the potential for an adverse outcome increases.[1,2,32]

AGENTS AVAILABLE FOR SEDATION OF ADOLESCENT PATIENTS
Nitrous Oxide/Oxygen Sedation

Short-term exposure to nitrous oxide induces sedation, euphoria, giddiness, elation, and a general sense of well-being. The pharmacologic mechanism of action of nitrous oxide is not fully understood. Multiple mechanisms are accepted. Nitrous oxide modulates ligand-gated ion channels, with activity on the gamma-aminobutyric acid type A (GABA-A) receptor and the N-methyl-d-aspartate (NMDA) receptor. Anxiolysis is the result of activation of the GABA-A receptor either directly or indirectly through at the benzodiazepine binding site.[33,34] The sedation/anesthetic, hallucinogenic, and euphoriant effects are likely caused by inhibition of NMDA-mediated currents.[35–37] Analgesic effects are linked to endogenous opioids and the noradrenergic systems.[33]

Nitrous oxide is the least potent of the inhalation anesthetics, but in dentistry, it is the most frequently used.[7] The minimum alveolar concentration of an agent that prevents movement in 50% of patients to a surgical incision for nitrous oxide is 105%. It is difficult to reach this level unless administered under hyperbaric conditions.[7] However,

Guedel's stage 2, delirium, can be reached if nitrous oxide is not properly administered.[8,9] Nitrous oxide may be administered alone or in combination with other agents.

There are relatively few absolute contraindications to nitrous oxide.[37] Fail-safe mechanisms prevent the percentage of oxygen from going below 30%. *Relative* contraindications to nitrous oxide include the following[33]:

- Chronic obstructive pulmonary disease
- Upper respiratory tract infections
- Middle ear/sinus disease
- Emotional disturbances or drug-related dependencies
- Pregnancy
- Treatment with bleomycin sulfate
- Methylenetetrahydrofolate reductase deficiency
- Cobalamin (vitamin B12) deficiency

Clinical Consideration:

Nitrous oxide/oxygen inhalation effectively reduces anxiety, produces analgesia, and enhances communication for adolescent dental patients.[33]

The following was excerpted from the *Handbook of Nitrous Oxide and Oxygen Sedation* by Clark and Brunick.[37] It is a good checklist when using nitrous oxide analgesia.

- Be enthusiastic and confident about the experience.
- Have confidence. Also, be knowledgeable about the limitations.
- Recognize that patients in your care represent the best opportunity you have to express genuine care and concern.
- Obtain informed consent before N_2O/O_2 administration.
- Practice titration.
- Start and end with 100% oxygen.
- Do not leave the patient alone.
- Document all procedures, reactions, complications, and so forth in the patient's record.
- Place patient in a comfortable position before administration.
- Inform the patient to ask for assistance at any time, if needed.
- If nitrous oxide is planned for the next visit, recommend not having a large meal before their appointment.

"Titrate to the level of sedation that is determined by patient comfort and relaxation. There is no percentage for sedation for a given experience or patient. There is also no pre-set liters per minute of nitrous oxide/oxygen. The percentage of nitrous oxide/oxygen given to a patient or experience will not reflect the amount necessary for any other experience. The goal is to keep the patient relaxed and comfortable."[37]

During emergence from nitrous oxide, the patient should return to his/her original emotional state. Terminate nitrous oxide flow; continue delivering 100% oxygen during the final minutes of the procedure. This begins the postoperative oxygenation phase of 3 to 5 minutes. Following this period, the patient should be recovered from the pharmacologic effects.[38]

N_2O/O_2 sedation may augment or balance other modalities of sedation and anesthesia. This can add safety because the patient is getting a minimum of 30% oxygen, which is greater than the 21% of room air. However, some states do not allow

| **Box 1** |
| **Potential adverse effects of nitrous oxide/oxygen analgesia** |
| Diffusion hypoxia |
| Nausea/vomiting |
| Postprocedure memory "fogginess" |
| Coordination/balance impairment |

polypharmacy, so augmentation may not be an option. **Box 1** lists potential adverse effects of nitrous oxide analgesia.

Benzodiazepines

Benzodiazepines bind the GABA-A receptor, increasing the frequency of the opening of the associated chloride channel. GABA-A is responsible for inhibition of CNS function, mainly in the thalamus and limbic systems, the area of the brain responsible for emotion and behavior. Benzodiazepines induce anxiolysis and sedation. Some agents are classified as anxiolytics, and others are classified as sedatives depending on their affinity for the GABA-A subunit.[7]

Benzodiazepines are the most popular and widely used sedative agents in dentistry. They are reversible with flumazenil and have a wide safety margin (therapeutic dose to toxic dose), making them desirable for sedation in dentistry.[7]

Midazolam (Dormicum or Versed), a short-acting, water-soluble benzodiazepine, is perhaps the most popular, versatile agent. It is often referred to as the mainstay of moderate sedation in dentistry.[39,40] This agent causes sedation with anterograde amnesia and has a relatively short half-life, which can be reversed.[41,42]

Midazolam and its routes of administration[7]:

1. *IM:* not well accepted and should be reserved for difficult patients, peaks in 15 minutes.
2. *IV:* venous access required. Smaller therapeutic index. Caution when used with opioids: respiratory depression may result/occur.
3. *Oral:* most popular pediatric route but difficult to mask bitter taste. Optimal separation from parents in 30 to 45 minutes. Dose: 0.5 mg/kg up to total of 20 mg maximum.
4. *Rectal:* most often use in diaper-age patients. Maximum plasma level is in 19 to 29 minutes. Disadvantages include variation in absorption and defecation.
5. *Nasal:* acidic solution that burns. May be poorly absorbed in cases of upper respiratory infections with increased nasal secretions. Sedation occurs in 7 to 10 minutes.

Paradoxic disinhibition has also been observed with benzodiazepines.[43] These reactions may include increased talkativeness, emotional release, hostility, impulsivity excitement, and excessive movement. Paradoxic reactions may occur in some patients with substance use disorders when compared with other groups. Most paradoxic reactions are idiosyncratic.[43] However, there is evidence to suggest these reactions may occur secondary to a genetic link, history of alcohol abuse, or psychological disturbances.[43–45] **Box 2** lists common adverse effects seen with benzodiazepines.

Clinical Consideration:

Benzodiazepines have a wide safety margin and a reversal agent. They are good options for sedation of the adolescent dental patient.

Flumazenil or Romazicon is the reversal agent for benzodiazepines. The agent is given via IV bolus (0.01–0.02 mg/kg maximum: 0.2 mg) and titrated to effect. The dentist may repeat at 1-minute intervals not to exceed a cumulative dose of 0.05 mg/kg or 1 mg, whichever is lower.[46] Lack of response after cumulative doses implies the cause of sedation is unlikely from benzodiazepines.[7] Sublingual administration of flumazenil is extremely controversial with few studies having been performed to evaluate efficacy.[47] Fluid boluses given under the tongue could cause edema and airway obstruction.[47]

Clinical Considerations:

Practitioners should recognize the half-life of flumazenil may be shorter than the benzodiazepine that is being reversed. Patients should be evaluated frequently for "relapse" of sedation or respiratory depression.

Caution should also be used when administering flumazenil to patients receiving chronic benzodiazepines because complete reversal may induce significant withdrawal symptoms and possible seizures.

Opioids

Opioids produce analgesia, sedation, anxiolysis, and respiratory depression. Opioids are used as strong analgesics, for the relief of moderate to severe pain.[7] Opioid analgesics are divided into 3 categories: (1) opioid agonists, (2) opioid agonist-antagonist, and (3) opioid antagonists. Opioid agonists interact with the receptors (mu, kappa, sigma, and delta) and produce a physiologic change.[48,49] Opioid antagonists when bound produce no pharmacologic effect. Mixed agents produce characteristics of both. The receptor activated will determine the physiologic effect, which may include analgesia, sedation, euphoria, dysphoria, and respiratory depression.[49]

Many opioid agonists are used for sedation (moderate and deep) in dentistry. Meperidine (Demerol) was one of the commonly used opioids in dentistry. It has been replaced by newer, safer agents like fentanyl and morphine, which have fewer side effects.[7] Meperidine's anticholinergic properties cause increased heart rate, dry mouth, and localized histamine (H1) release.[50] These properties are not seen with the newer agents.

Box 2
Common adverse effects with benzodiazepines

Oversedation

Mild postprocedure amnesia

Respiratory depression

Drowsiness

Coordination-balance difficulties

Paradoxic reactions

Morphine is the gold standard, by which other opioid agonists are compared for strength. Morphine's longer duration of action makes it less desirable for outpatient dental surgery under sedation or anesthesia. Fentanyl, 100 times more potent than morphine, may be a better option because of its rapid onset and short duration of action.[51] Analgesia and sedation are immediate with IV fentanyl with the maximum effect observed in approximately 2 to 3 minutes.[51]

Relative contraindications to the use of opioid agonists include patients under 2 years old, pregnant patients, patients with recent history of head trauma or CNS-related pathologic condition, and patients who were administered monoamine oxidase inhibitors within the past 14 days. Caution must be used in patients with renal or liver dysfunction. Decreased metabolism and clearance could result in opioid overdose.[7] Opioids also cause respiratory depression and stiff chest syndrome, which may result in hypoventilation and hypoxia. *Dentists who administer opioids must be able to administer positive pressure ventilation when indicated.*[3]

Opioids are reversed with a pure opioid antagonist, naloxone hydrochloride.[48] IV administration should result in rapid reversal of respiratory depression, and sedative effects. Naloxone's duration of action is approximately 20 to 30 minutes; resedation may occur if long-acting agonists are reversed. Reversal agents should be administered with care to persons with known or suspected physical dependence on opioids. Abrupt or complete reversal may result in "acute abstinence syndrome."[7]

Opioid abuse in adolescent patients is a real concern. Over the previous decades, self-reported use of heroin and nonmedical use of prescription opioids have increased.[52] Increased availability of highly addictive prescription opioids makes this a frequently abused drug.[52] Users of opioids are at increased risk for drug overdose, drug dependence, and mental health disorders. This group, also, has increased risk for developing blood-borne viral infections, either through sharing of injection equipment or through unsafe sexual activities performed under the influence.[52]

Common adverse events of opioids are listed in **Box 3**.

Clinical considerations:
Opioids are indicated for painful procedures. Opioid administration requires physiologic monitoring and continuous observation.

Ketamine

Ketamine hydrochloride, a dissociative anesthetic, is an NMDA receptor antagonist.[53] Patients appear awake, but unaware of, or dissociated from the environment.[54] It is commonly used in pediatric anesthesia and patients with developmental disabilities. Routinely it is given with benzodiazepines to provide amnesia and analgesia. Ketamine produces little to no respiratory depression as compared with benzodiazepines and

---

Box 3
Common adverse effects of opioids

Sedation

Respiratory depression/apnea

Constipation

Dizziness

Confusion

opioids. It increases heart rate, blood pressure, and intracranial pressure. Nystagmus and an incompetent gag reflex are also observed. Copious secretions are a result of ketamine administration and must be aggressively managed to prevent laryngospasm.[54]

There is no reversal agent for ketamine; therefore, the dentist must be prepared to manage the patient and their level of sedation. Different states have different guidelines for the use of ketamine for sedation in the dental office.

Common adverse effects of ketamine are listed in **Box 4**.

Propofol

Propofol is a nonbenzodiazepine, nonbarbiturate anesthetic, originally designed as an induction agent for general anesthesia.[55] Sleep is induced through potentiation of the GABA receptor slowing the channel's closing time.[56] Propofol is popular in outpatient venues because of its sedation properties.[57] Subhypnotic doses produce excellent sedation with minimal respiratory depression and short recovery periods.[7] Propofol should only be administered by providers with anesthesia training.[55]

Common adverse effects of propofol are listed in **Box 5**.

Antihistamines

H1 blockers are used in the treatment of allergic reactions, in drying of secretions, and as mild anxiolysis/sedation. A side effect of the histamines is CNS depression or sedation.[58] Antihistamines carry a wide therapeutic window and high margin of safety, making them popular in sedation dentistry.[7]

Hydroxyzine, a diphenylmethane, is perhaps the most widely used antihistamine in pediatric dentistry.[59,60] It may be administered as a solo agent for management of patients with mild to moderate fear. Combinations of hydroxyzine and other drugs, such as meperidine and midazolam, are used for patients who require deeper levels of sedation.[61]

Antihistamines, like benzodiazepines, may cause paradoxic reactions in young children, adults with genetic predisposition, and individuals with psychiatric and/or personality disorders.[43] Comorbid psychiatric conditions predispose to idiosyncratic reactions.[62] Therefore, management of the psychiatric illness may reduce the severity of the paradoxic reaction. Common adverse reactions to H1 antagonists are listed in **Box 6**.

Alpha Agonists

Precedex or dexmedetomidine is an α_2 agonist indicated for sedation. Because dexmedetomidine exerts its effects via the α_2-adrenoceptor, it has a different mechanism of action than its GABA-mimetics, such as propofol or benzodiazepines.[63] The sedative effects of dexmedetomidine are mediated by the α_2-adrenergic receptor, a G-protein–coupled receptor. Activation in the brain and spinal cord inhibits neuronal firing, causing hypotension, bradycardia, sedation, and analgesia. The presynaptic receptor

---

Box 4
Common adverse effects of ketamine

Emergence agitation

Increased salivation

Tachycardia

Box 5
Common adverse effects of propofol

Hypotension

Respiratory depression/apnea

Injection site reaction

Phlebitis

---

inhibits the release of norepinephrine, terminating the propagation of pain signals. Postsynaptic activation of α_2 receptors inhibits sympathetic activity, which decreases blood pressure and heart rate.

Studies show the level of sedation with dexmedetomidine was comparable to that of midazolam and better than lorazepam.[64] It was also shown to have less delirium and tachycardia.[65] Dexmedetomidine mimics natural sleep and does not depress respiration.[63]

Inhalation Anesthetics and Neuromuscular Blocking Agents

Inhalation anesthetics are used for general anesthesia.[7] These agents provide maintenance of general anesthesia and are nontoxic to the organ systems. Sevoflurane, isoflurane, and desflurane are the mainstay of inhalation anesthetics. Sevoflurane is also indicated for mask induction of general anesthesia.[66]

Muscle relaxants or neuromuscular-blocking drugs provide skeletal muscle relaxation to facilitate tracheal intubation and mechanical ventilation.[7] There are 2 types of muscle relaxants: depolarizing muscle relaxants (succinylcholine) and nondepolarizing muscle relaxants (eg, atracurium, vecuronium, rocuronium, pancuronium). Neuromuscular blocking agents impair respiratory function and cause apnea. Succinylcholine may be used in the treatment of laryngospasm.[3]

Local Anesthetics

Local anesthetics are cardiac depressants and may cause CNS excitation or depression.[3] The sedative effects of local anesthetics are enhanced when used at higher doses and in combination with opioids. Therefore, it is paramount not to exceed the maximum allowable safe dosage.[3] Common adverse reactions to local anesthetics are listed in **Box 7**.

Clinical Consideration:

It is recommended that the dentist calculate the dose (mg/kg) before administration and administer slowly and with frequent aspiration to avoid possible intravascular injection.

Box 6
Common adverse effects of histamine antagonists

Anticholinergic (dry eyes, urinary retention, dry mouth, constipation)

> **Box 7**
> **Common adverse reactions or complications to local anesthetics**
>
> Hypersensitivity reactions
>
> Vascular administration
>
> Injection site pain postprocedure

BALANCED TECHNIQUE

Balanced anesthesia is a concept designed to minimize risk and maximize benefit. A balanced protocol requires assessment of the adolescent patient and the procedure. The technique pairs decreased dosages of concurrent mixtures to summate the goals of a desired sedation/anesthetic.

MONITORING AND DOCUMENTATION

Studies show that routine application of minimal monitors enables the detection of subtle physiologic changes, which permit measures to be taken before there is a catastrophic event.[67] A national standard now exists for intraoperative monitoring.[68] As a rule of thumb, the deeper the sedation, the more aggressive the monitoring.[68,69]

EMERGENCIES

The standards of care for sedation-related emergencies are the same as for any medical emergency. Recognition and action are key steps. Dentists who treat using local anesthesia alone see syncope as a medical emergency. Dentists who administer moderate sedation occasionally experience unconsciousness or apnea and should be prepared to treat the patient seamlessly. Deep sedation and general anesthesia render the patient unconscious, so apnea is a routine occurrence and would not be considered an emergency. What may be an emergency to one provider is a normal occurrence to another.[7] Risk versus benefit analysis specific to each adolescent patient will help prevent medical emergencies.

Dentists should have a comfortable relationship with the patient, their family, and their medical providers. They should use familiar drugs and techniques, limit the use to patients who require them, have a comprehensive preoperative evaluation, and use continuous monitoring all in an effort to minimize sedation-related events. An emergency system should be in place with well-trained personnel who can follow protocol. *High-risk patients should be treated in a hospital setting.*[3]

It is vital that the dentist is familiar with indications, contraindications, dosages, and methods of administration of emergency drugs. They should also have appropriately sized equipment and be able to correctly operate it.

Potential emergency situations include the following[3,7,46]:

1. Apnea
2. Airway obstruction
3. Laryngospasm
4. Pulmonary aspiration
5. Desaturation
6. Overdose
7. Hyperventilation
8. Allergic reactions

9. Cardiac arrhythmias
10. Seizures
11. Hypoglycemia

Once an emergency has been identified, remain calm; assess the situation and follow the *PABCDE's*[7]:

P = Position: Always position patient appropriately
A = Airway: Assess airway is patency
B = Breathing: Determine if patient is breathing
C = Circulation: Check the pulse
D = Definitive care: May include activation of EMS and establishing IV access
E = Electricity: Assess need

Clinical Considerations:
Respiratory events are a common cause of sedation-related emergencies in pediatric patients with normal cardiac function. Therefore, the dentist must have airway management skills and be proficient with positive pressure ventilation (bag-valve-mask) with 100% oxygen. When airway issues are not addressed, the respiratory event could result in cardiac arrest.

Special Considerations

Obesity

Adolescent and childhood obesity has reached epidemic levels in the United States.[70] In some reports, about 17% of children in the United States are obese.[70] According to the Centers for Disease Control and Prevention (CDC), the prevalence of obesity is 19.3% (4.4 million children and adolescents).[71] Hispanic and non-Hispanic black children have the highest rates of obesity.[71] Body mass index (BMI) and the CDC's normative BMI percentiles are used to diagnose overweight and obesity in children and adolescents.[72] A BMI ≥85th percentile but less than 95th percentile for age and sex is considered overweight, whereas ≥95th percentile is considered obese.[72] The CDC suggests checking the BMI at least annually during well and/or sick visits.

Some adolescents are diagnosed with syndromes associated with genetic obesity with or without developmental delay. Examples of these are Prader Willi, Albright, SIM1 deficiency, and Alstrom and Leptin deficiency. o The risk and benefits should be considered carefully when sedation is intended.[72] These conditions may not be conducive for moderate sedation.

The provision of inhalation sedation with nitrous oxide during which oxygen levels are maintained at or above 30% may be more appropriate.[73] If IV sedation is proposed, the overall benefit to the patient must be carefully weighed against the increased likelihood of significant respiratory depression and the difficulties in managing a respiratory complication.[73] Opioids, especially in large doses, should be avoided because of their greater likelihood of producing respiratory compromise.[74] Triazolam, a short-acting benzodiazepine with inactive metabolites, can be considered. The recommended dosage range is 0.125 to 0.25 mg.[75] Midazolam, a popular drug used for pediatric oral sedation, offers no advantage over triazolam.[76] Judicious administration of local anesthetics during sedation must also be followed. Multiple use of medications, coupled with sedatives, can result in synergism, which can easily potentiate the sedative effects on the patient. Prolonged somnolence and paradoxic reactions can occur because of slow distribution of sedatives. Therefore, proper recovery and discharge must be adhered to for patient safety.

Attention-deficit/hyperactivity disorder

Attention-deficit/hyperactivity disorder (ADHD) is one of the most common childhood disorders and can continue through adolescence and into adulthood.[77] The CDC estimates around 2 to 3 million adolescents in 2016 are diagnosed, with increasing prevalence.[78] ADHD is marked by a consistent pattern of inattention and/or hyperactivity-impulsivity that interferes with daily life functions and development.[77] Symptoms can change as the child grows into adolescence. However, inattention, restlessness, and impulsivity tend to continue into adulthood.[77]

Treatment and therapies are aimed to control the symptoms and improve the quality of life and self-esteem of the adolescent. Medications commonly used to treat ADHD symptoms include stimulants, such as methylphenidate and amphetamine; nonstimulants, such as atomoxetine; tricyclic antidepressants; and alpha agonists.[79] Psychotherapy, stress management, and support groups are nonpharmacologic modalities used. Anxiety disorder is a comorbidity of ADHD, which can manifest in the dental setting.[80]

The most frequently used mode of sedation for these patients is nitrous oxide analgesia with a high success rate.[81,82] Benzodiazepines, such as diazepam, in combination with nitrous oxide are also used.[81] Midazolam, a frequently used sedative in pediatric dentistry, can cause untoward paradoxic reactions.[83] Other medications, such as α_2-adrenergic receptor agonists like clonidine, tizanidine, and dexmedetomidine, have also been used.[84] Sedation adverse events are less likely if patients are accustomed to the dose of their medication.[85] It is also imperative for patients to take their prescribed medication the day of sedation. IV sedation or general anesthesia may be in indicated for individuals with extreme anxiety.

SUMMARY

There are many modalities to control pain and anxiety in adolescent dental patients. The method of choice should be exclusively based on risk versus benefit, the provider's comfort level and training, and the patient's needs. The challenge is keeping balance between enough and too much. This is accomplished by choosing agents that meet the patient's needs (antianxiety, pain control, or sedation). There is no one correct method for each patient or provider. No panacea exists, nor is one technique going to work for every adolescent patient. Therefore, having multiple options will decrease risk of failure.

CLINICS CARE POINTS

- Sedation and Anesthesia may be used to manage pain/anxiety and modify behavior to safely complete dental procedures in adolescent patients.
- Sedation and anesthesia occur along a continuum, practitioners must anticipate the level of sedation and be prepared to diagnose and manage the physiologic consequences of patients whose level is deeper than initially intended.
- The sedation/anesthetic regimen for adolescent dental patients should have a high therapeutic index with a wide safety margin and a low probability for abuse.
- Nitrous oxide/oxygen inhalation is a safe and effective agent which reduces anxiety, produces analgesia, and enhances communication for adolescent dental patients.

DISCLAIMER

This article is not intended to make you proficient in sedation for the adolescent dental patient. Information presented is based on Guidelines from the American Academy of

Pediatric Dentistry (AAPD), American Dental Association (ADA), American Association of Pediatrics (AAP), and the American Society of Anesthesiologists (ASA). Practitioners are required to know state guidelines before administering any type of sedation.

RESOURCES AND FURTHER READINGS

Available at: http://www.ada.org/~/media/ADA/Advocacy/Files/anesthesia_use_guidelines.pdf.

DISCLOSURE

The authors have nothing to disclose.

REFERENCES

1. Excerpted from Continuum of Depth of Sedation: definition of general anesthesia and levels of sedation/analgesia, 2014, of the American Society of Anesthesiologists. A copy of the full text can be obtained from ASA, 1061 American Lane Schaumburg, IL 60173-4973. Available at: www.asahq.org%20. Accessed April 25, 2021.
2. American Society of Anesthesiologists Task Force on Sedation and Analgesia by Non-Anesthesiologists: practice guidelines for sedation and analgesia by non-anesthesiologists. Anesthesiology 2002;96:1004–17.
3. Coté CJ, Wilson S. American Academy of Pediatric Dentistry, American Academy of Pediatrics. Guidelines for Monitoring and Management of Pediatric Patients Before, During, and After Sedation for Diagnostic and Therapeutic Procedures. Pediatric Dent 2019;41(4):E26–52.
4. American Dental Association, Council on Dental Education and Licensure. Guidelines for teaching pediatric pain control and sedation to dentists and dental students. As adopted by the January 2021 ADA House of Delegates. Chicago: The Association; 2021.
5. American Dental Association, Council on Dental Education. Guidelines for the use of sedation and general anesthesia by dentists. As adopted by the Oct. 2016 ADA House of Delegates. Chicago: The Association; 2016.
6. American Dental Association, Council on Dental Education. Guidelines for teaching pain control and sedation to dentists and dental students. As adopted by the Oct. 2016 ADA House of Delegates. Chicago: The Association; 2016.
7. Malamed SF. Sedation: a guide to patient management. 6th edition. St. Louis (MO): Mosby Elsevier; 2017.
8. Douglas BL. A re-evaluation of Guedel's stages of anesthesia: with particular reference to the ambulatory dental patient. J Am Dent Soc Anesthesiol 1958; 5:11–4.
9. Harrison-Calmes S. Arthur Guedel, M.D., and the eye signs of anesthesia. Am Soc Anesthesiologists, Newsletter 2002;66.
10. Cote CJ, Notterman DS, Karl HW, et al. Adverse sedation events in pediatrics: a critical incident analysis of contributory factors. Pediatrics 2000;105:805–14.
11. Hoffman GM, Nowakowski R, Troshynski TJ, et al. Risk reduction in pediatric procedural sedation by application of an American Academy of Pediatrics/American Society of Anesthesiologists process model. Pediatrics 2002;109:236–43.
12. Kennedy RM, Luchman JD. he "ouchless emergency department." Getting closer: advances in decreasing distress during painful procedures in the emergency department. Pediatr Clin North Am 1999;46:1215–47.

13. Fleisher LA, Beckman JA, Brown KA, et al. ACC/AHA 2007 guidelines on perioperative cardiovascular evaluation and care for noncardiac surgery: executive summary. Circulation 2007;116:1971–96.

14. Eagle KA, Berger PB, Calkins H, et al. ACC/AHA guideline update for perioperative cardiovascular evaluation for noncardiac surgery—executive summary a report of the American College of Cardiology/American Heart Association Task Force on Practice Guidelines (Committee to Update the 1996 Guidelines on Perioperative Cardiovascular Evaluation for Noncardiac Surgery). Circulation 2002; 105:1257–67.

15. American Society of Anesthesiologist. New classification of physical status. Anesthesiology 1963;24:111.

16. Preoperative Assessment, Premedication, & Perioperative Documentation. In: Butterworth J, MacKay D, Wasnick J, editors. Morgan Mikhail's Clinical Anesthesiology. 6th Edition. New York: Mc-Graw Hill Education; 2018. p. 295–7.

17. Lagasse RS. Anesthesia safety: model of myth? A review of published literature and analysis of current original data. Anesthesiology 2002;97:1609–17.

18. Malviya S, Vopel-Lewis T, Tait AR. Adverse events and risk factors associated with the sedation of children by non-anesthesiologist. Anesth Analg 1997;85: 1207–13.

19. Carr MP, Horton JE. Clinical evaluation and comparison of 2 topical anesthetics for pain caused by needle sticks and scaling and root planing. J Periodontol 2001;72(4):479–84.

20. Fukota O, Braham RL, Yanase H, et al. The sedative effect of intranasal midazolam administration in the dental treatment of patients with mental disabilities. Part 1. The effect of 0.2 mg/kg dose. J Clin Pediatr Dent 1993;17(4):231–7.

21. Fuks AB, Kaufman E, Ram D, et al. Assessment of two doses of intranasal midazolam for sedation of pediatric dental patients. Pediatr Dent 1994;16(4):301–5.

22. Lam C, Udin RD, Malamed SF, et al. Midazolam premedication in children: a pilot study comparing intramuscular and intranasal administration. Anesth Prog 2005; 52(2):56–61.

23. Walbergh EJ, Wills RJ, Eckhert J. Plasma concentrations of midazolam in children following intranasal administration. Anesthesiology 1991;74:233.

24. Jastak JT, Donaldson D. Nitrous oxide. Anesth Prog 1991;38:172.

25. Sinner B, Graf BM. Ketamine. Handbook Exp Pharmacol 2008;(182):313–33.

26. Mace SE, Barata IA, Cravero JP, et al. Clinical policy: evidence-based approach to pharmacologic agents used in pediatric sedation and analgesia in the emergency department. Ann Emerg Med 2004;44:342–77.

27. Deshpande JK, Tobias JD, editors. The pediatric pain handbook. St. Louis (MO): Mosby; 1996.

28. Alcaino EA. Conscious sedation in paediatric dentistry: current philosophies and techniques. Ann R Australas Coll Dent Surg 2000;15:206–10.

29. Yaster M, Krane EJ, Kaplan RF, et al, editors. Pediatric pain management and sedation handbook. St Louis (MO): Mosby; 1997.

30. Cravero CH, Notterman DS, Karl HW, et al. Review of pediatric sedation. Anesth Analg 2004;99:1355–64.

31. Krauss B, Green SM. Procedural sedation and analgesia in children. Lancet 2006;367:766–80.

32. Mitchell AA, Louik C, Lacouture P, et al. Risks to children from computed tomographic scan premedication. JAMA 1982;247:2385–8.

33. American Academy of Pediatric Dentistry. Use of nitrous oxide for pediatric dental patients, . The reference manual of pediatric dentistry. Chicago, Ill: American Academy of Pediatric Dentistry; 2020. p. 324–9.

34. Emmanouil DE, Quock RM. Advances in understanding the actions of nitrous oxide. Anesth Prog 2007;54(1):9–18.

35. Yamakura T, Harris RA. Effects of gaseous anaesthetics nitrous oxide and xenon on ligand-gated ion channels. Comparison with isoflurane and ethanol. Anesthesiology 2000;93(4):1095–101.

36. Mennerick S, Jevtovic-Todorovic V, Todorovic SM, et al. Effect of nitrous oxide on excitatory and inhibitory synaptic transmission in hippocampal cultures. J Neurosci 1998;18(23):9716–26.

37. Clark MS, Brunick AL. Handbook of nitrous oxide and oxygen sedation. 5th edition. St Louis (MO): Mosby; 2019.

38. Jastak JT, Orendruff D. Recovery from nitrous. sedation" Anesth Prog 1975;22: 113–6.

39. Parnis SJ, Foate JA, Vander Wlath JH, et al. "Oral midazolam is an effective premedication for children having day-stay anaesthesia. Anaesth Intensive Care 1992;20:9–14.

40. Feld LH, Negus JB, White PF. Oral midazolam preanesthetic drug in pediatric outpatients. Anesthesiology 1990;73:831.

41. Conner JT, Katz RL, Pagano RR, et al. Midazolam for intravenous surgical premedication, and induction of general anesthesia. Anesth Analg 1978;57:1.

42. Hennesy MJ, Kirby KC, Montgomery IM. Comparison of the amnesic effects of midazolam and diazepam. Psychopharmacology 1991;103:545.

43. Carissa E, Mancuso CE, Tanzi MG, et al. Paradoxical reactions to benzodiazepines: literature review and treatment options. Pharmacotherapy 2004;24(9): 1177–85.

44. Weinbroum AA, Szold O, Ogorek D, et al. The midazolam-induced paradox phenomenon is reversible by flumazenil: epidemiology, patient characteristics and review of the literature. Eur J Anaesthesiol 2001;18:789–97.

45. Short TG, Forrest P, Galletly DC. Paradoxical reactions to benzodiazepines: a genetically determined phenomenon? Anaesth Intens Care 1987;15:330–45.

46. American Academy of Pediatric Dentistry. Management of medical emergencies" the reference manual of pediatric dentistry. Chicago Ill: American Academy of Pediatric Dentistry; 2020. p. 600–1.

47. Hosaka K, Jackson D, Pickrell JE, et al. Flumazenil reversal of sublingual triazolam: a randomized controlled clinical trial. J Am Dent Assoc 2009;140(No 5): 559–66.

48. Martin WR. Naloxone. Ann Intern Med 1976;85:765.

49. Dahan A, Niesters, M, Olofsen E, et al. Editors. Clinical Anesthesia 7th Edition. Philadelphia: Lippincott Williams & Wilkins; 2013. p. 502–22.

50. Pallasch TJ. Clinical drug therapy in dental practice. Philadelphia: Lea & Febiger; 1973.

51. Wedell D, Hersh EV. A review of the opioid analgesics. Fentanyl Alfentanil Sufentanil Compend 1991;12:184–7.

52. Bryson EO. The anesthetic implications of illicit opioid use. Int Anesthesiol Clin 2011;49(1):67–78.

53. Reich DL, Silvay G. Ketamine: an update on the first twenty-five years of clinical experience. Can J Anaesth 1989;36:186.

54. Haas DA, Harper DG. Ketamine: a review of its pharmacologic properties and use in ambulatory anesthesia. Anesth Prog 1992;39:61.

55. Stuart Pharmaceuticals, Diprivan. Drug package insert. Wilmington, Delaware: Stuart Pharmaceuticals; 1992.
56. Trapani G, Altomare C, Liso G, et al. Propofol in anesthesia. Mechanism of action, structure-activity relationships, and drug delivery. Curr Med Chem 2000;7(2): 249–71.
57. MacKenzie N, Grant IS. Propofol for intravenous sedation. Anaesthesia 1987; 42:3.
58. Richardson GS, Roehrs TA, Rosenthal L, et al. Tolerance to daytime sedative effects of H1 antihistamines. J Clin Psychopharmacol 2002;22(5):511–5.
59. Wright GZ, Chiasson RC. Current premedicating trends in pedodontics. ASDC J Dent Child 1973;40:185.
60. Wright GZ, Chiasson RC. The use of sedation drugs by Canadian pediatric dentists. Pediatr Dent 1987;9:308.
61. Torres-Perez J, Tapia-Garcia I, Rosales-Berber MA, et al. Comparison of three conscious sedation regimens for pediatric dental patients. J Clin Pediatr Dent 2007;31(3):183–6.
62. Antochi R, Stavarkaki C, Emery PC. Psychopharmacological treatments in persons with dual diagnosis of psychiatric disorders and developmental disabilities. Postgrad Med J 2003;79:139–46.
63. Hospira: Precedex. Drug package insert. Lake Forest, IL: Hospira, Inc; 2012.
64. Riker RR, Shehabi Y, Bokesch PM, et al. Dexmedetomidine vs midazolam for sedation of critically ill patients: a randomized trial. JAMA 2009;301(5):489–99.
65. Pandharipande PP, Pun BT, Herr DL, et al. Effect of sedation with dexmedetomidine vs lorazepam on acute brain dysfunction in mechanically ventilated patients: the MENDS randomized controlled trial. JAMA 2007;298(22):2644–53.
66. Abbott. ULTANE® (sevoflurane) volatile liquid for inhalation. North Chicago, IL: Abbott Laboratories; 2003. Drug Package Insert.
67. Emergency Care Research Institute. Death during general anesthesia. J Health Care Technol 1985;1:155.
68. Standards for basic intra-operative monitoring. ASA Newsl 1986;50:13.
69. Hart LS, Berns SD, Houck CS, et al. The value of end-tidal CO_2 monitoring when comparing three methods of conscious sedation for children undergoing painful procedure in the emergency department. Pediatr Emerg Care 1997;13:189–93.
70. Sanyaolu A, Okorie C, Qi X, et al. Childhood and adolescent obesity in the United States: a public health concern. Glob Pediatr Health 2019;6. 2333794X19891305.
71. Fryar CD, Carroll MD, Afful J. Prevalence of overweight, obesity, and severe obesity among children and adolescents aged 2–19 years: United States, 1963–1965 through 2017–2018. NCHS Health E-Stats; 2020.
72. Styne DM, Arslanian SA, Connor EL, et al. Pediatric obesity-assessment, treatment, and prevention: an endocrine society clinical practice guideline. J Clin Endocrinol Metab 2017;102(3):709–57.
73. Reilly D, Boyle C, Craig D. Obesity and dentistry: a growing problem. Br Dent J 2009;207:171–5.
74. Baker S, Yagiela J. Obesity: a complicating factor for sedation in children. Pediatr Dent 2006;28 6:487–93.
75. Weaver JM. When can a normal dose be an overdose? Who is at risk? Anesth Prog 2014;61(2):45–6.
76. Donaldson M, Gizzarelli G, Chanpong B. Oral sedation: a primer on anxiolysis for the adult patient. Anesth Prog 2007;54(3):118–29.
77. National Institute of Mental Health. Available at: www.nimh.nih.gov. Accessed April 25, 2021.

78. Centers for Disease Control. Available at: www.cdc.gov. Accessed April 25, 2021.
79. Osland ST, Steeves TD, Pringsheim T. Pharmacological treatment for attention deficit hyperactivity disorder (ADHD) in children with comorbid tic disorders. Cochrane Database Syst Rev 2018;6(6):CD007990.
80. Reale L, Bartoli B, Cartabia M, et al, Lombardy ADHD Group. Comorbidity prevalence and treatment outcome in children and adolescents with ADHD. Eur Child Adolesc Psychiatry 2017;26(12):1443–57.
81. Kerins CA, McWhorter AG, Seale NS. Pharmacologic behavior management of pediatric dental patients diagnosed with attention deficit disorder/attention deficit hyperactivity disorder. Pediatr Dent 2007;29(6):507–13.
82. Chi SI, Kim H, Seo KS. Analysis of application of dental sedation in attention deficit hyperactivity disorder (ADHD) patients using the Korean National Health Insurance data. J Dent Anesth Pain Med 2021;21(2):99–111.
83. Marshall WR, Weaver BD, McCutcheon P. A study of the effectiveness of oral midazolam as a dental pre-operative sedative and hypnotic. Spec Care Dentist 1999; 19(6):259–66.
84. Giovannitti JA Jr, Thoms SM, Crawford JJ. Alpha-2 adrenergic receptor agonists: a review of current clinical applications. Anesth Prog 2015;62(1):31–9.
85. Faraone SV, Glatt SJ. Effects of extended-release guanfacine on ADHD symptoms and sedation-related adverse events in children with ADHD. J Atten Disord 2010;13(5):532–8.

Pediatric Endodontic Treatment of Adolescent Patients

Adriana Modesto Vieira, DDS, MS, PhD, DMD[a,b,c,*],
Herbert L. Ray Jr, DMD[d,e,f]

KEYWORDS

- Adolescents • Immature permanent teeth • Deep caries • Pulp • Pulp capping
- Pulpotomy

KEY POINTS

- Pulp therapy treatment in adolescent patients presents several challenges to clinicians, varying from pulpal diagnosis to restorability considerations for immature young permanent teeth with deep carious lesions or with dental defects approximating the pulp or traumatic dental injuries.
- Efforts should be made by clinicians to achieve completion of root formation in immature young permanent teeth and continued growth and development of the oral facial structures.
- Considerations of behavior guidance options, modification of techniques to account for incomplete root development, and the level of dental homecare must all be balanced when designing endodontic and restorative treatment plans for adolescent patients.
- Being able to provide treatment of this subpopulation is gratifying and critical in setting the path of oral health into adulthood for these patients.

INTRODUCTION

Endodontic treatment of adolescent patients does not present any special pulp therapy techniques. However, the considerations for using pulp therapy techniques that are routinely performed on mature patients become complex during early

[a] Department of Pediatric Dentistry, University of Pittsburgh School of Dental Medicine, 3501 Terrace Street, 366A Salk Hall, Pittsburgh, PA 15261, USA; [b] Office of Diversity, Inclusion and Social Justice, University of Pittsburgh School of Dental Medicine, Pittsburgh, PA, USA; [c] Department of Oral and Craniofacial Sciences, University of Pittsburgh School of Dental Medicine, Pittsburgh, PA, USA; [d] Department of Endodontics, University of Pittsburgh School of Dental Medicine, 3501 Terrace Street, 3063 Salk Annex, Pittsburgh, PA 15261, USA; [e] Center for Craniofacial Regeneration, University of Pittsburgh School of Dental Medicine, Pittsburgh, PA, USA; [f] McGowan Institute for Regenerative Medicine, University of Pittsburgh, 3025 East Carson Street, Pittsburgh, PA 15203, USA
* Corresponding author. Department of Pediatric Dentistry, University of Pittsburgh School of Dental Medicine, 3501 Terrace Street, 366A Salk Hall, Pittsburgh, PA 15261.
E-mail address: ams208@pitt.edu

Dent Clin N Am 65 (2021) 775–785
https://doi.org/10.1016/j.cden.2021.07.001
0011-8532/21/© 2021 Elsevier Inc. All rights reserved.

adolescence years. These considerations directly depend on unique factors such as the stage of tooth development, behavior assessment of the patient during the endodontic treatment, caregiver and patient's general attitude toward oral health, quality of home care, and other factors that interfere with the control of the pulp's inflammation and/or infection.

A study by Al-Madi and colleagues[1] found that 36.9% of children between the ages of 6 and 18 years required dental treatment that had pulpal involvement. Only 21.8% of the teeth received completed endodontic therapy. The remaining 59% only received temporary restorations and 24% resulted in extraction. It has been suggested that several factors interfered with completion of dental treatment and tooth survival.[1,2] The immediate placement of a permanent restorative material is required for achievement of high success rates after completion of vital pulp therapy.[3,4]

This article discusses the specific endodontic therapies that are available for the adolescent population according to the American Academy of Pediatric Dentistry and American Association of Endodontists.[5,6] A decision tree is provided to help guide clinicians through the steps to arrive at a therapy that will provide immediate relief for the patient while taking into consideration the future options for follow-up care for the patient when entering into adulthood. There are several factors that can affect the health of the dental pulp.[7,8] For the purpose of this article, the focus is primarily on the impact of bacteria being the primary concern, whether their entry was a result of dental caries, restorative procedures, trauma, or genetic conditions affecting the dentin pulp complex.

DENTAL PULP COMPLEX
Dental Pulp and Its Protective Nature

The dental pulp is composed of connective tissue and contains a large number of odontoblasts, fibroblasts, and undifferentiated mesenchymal stem cells that can be used for dentin and pulp regeneration.[9,10]

The dental pulp has a strong propensity for survival, and protection of the periapical tissues specifically.[11–13] The larger dentinal tubules of the young tooth permit greater access of microbial contaminants to communicate with the pulp. The first cell to respond is the odontoblast. As irritants reach the odontoblastic process, the odontoblast signals the first inflammatory response through the activation of Toll-like receptors , and nucleotide-binding oligomerization domain (NOD)–like receptors starting the cascade of inflammatory reactions leading to the deposition of reactionary and reparative dentin.[14] As the bacteria move closer to the pulp, the ensuing neurogenic inflammatory response leads to sprouting of free nerve endings releasing calcitonin gene–related peptide and substance P.[15,16] This process begins the localized inflammatory response at the pulp-dentin interface. Vascular changes follow and lead to increased pulp blood flow,[17] bringing an initial influx of proinflammatory cytokines to the damaged region. It has been shown that this localized inflammatory response is very limited, and tissue as close as several millimeters remains healthy.[18] The arteriovenous anastomosis and its shunts open and redirect pulpal blood flow away from the directly affected region, thus minimizing the spread of contaminants to larger portions of the dental pulp complex.[19] The large diameter of the root canal system of the adolescent tooth and the still-forming anatomic apices permit the rich vascularity of the maturing dental pulp. Maintaining this pulpal tissue permits not only the immunologic protection of the periapices but also the continued deposition of radicular dentin and root formation. The remaining vital pulp tissue prevents the egress of bacterial irritants through the dentinal tubules/accessory canals by the presence of a vital odontoblastic process and the outward flow of dentinal fluid because of the intrapulpal pressure related to vital pulp.

As these basic principles of pulp biology are considered, permitting vital tissues to remain in adolescent patients provides greater opportunity for future treatment if necessary and allows the innate protective function of the dental pulp to aid in long-term tooth survival.

Clinical Evaluation of Pulp Inflammation

Previous histologic studies have shown that there is no association between clinical signs or symptoms and pulp inflammation.[20–23] However, historically, when collecting evidence of mild or moderate pain, normal pulp vitality, and negative sign to percussion, clinicians have classified the pulp inflammation as reversible, whereas evidence of severe pain or history of pain associated or not with periapical radiolucency was designated as irreversible pulp inflammation with indication for endodontic therapy or extraction.[24]

More recently, there has been strong consensus in the endodontic literature that clinical evaluation of teeth (ie, pain quality and responses to pulp testing) only indicate the probable status of the dental pulp complex. As examples of limitations of the clinical pulpal status categorization currently used, teeth clinically diagnosed as having irreversible symptomatic pulpitis may not present with histologic deep inflammation; comparison, pulp necrosis may happen in asymptomatic patients who were diagnosed with a reversible pulp inflammation. In summary, clinical diagnosis of the dental pulp complex is not reliable, and the severity of pulp inflammation and the pulp's potential of responding to appropriate endodontic procedures cannot be accurately determined unless other strategies are used.[25–27]

HOW TO NAVIGATE FROM OPEN APICES TO COMPLETE ROOT FORMATION OF PERMANENT TEETH OF ADOLESCENT PATIENTS
Treatment Complexity and Team Approach

Management of pulp tissues of immature permanent teeth creates a special set of circumstances.[6,28,29] The age of the patient dictates specialized behavior guidance skills as well as proper treatment planning because of children's growth and development considerations. The skill level and various pulp therapies, from nonsurgical root canal therapy with or without placement of a calcium silicate cement biologic plug to partial/full pulpotomies, are best managed by a knowledgeable clinician and require adequate time to perform these procedures. Because of the nature of, and length of time to perform, most of these procedures, patients require treatment under some form of sedation, ranging from nitrous oxide to general anesthesia. This specialized care is best coordinated by a team approach of the pediatric dentist, endodontist, and dental anesthesiologist.

Pulp Therapy Treatment Options

The decision of which course of treatment to follow is arrived at through the objective clinical findings, the subjective clinical assessment, and the level of sedation required to manage the patient (**Fig. 1**). Conservative therapies are always the goal; however, the ability to perform emergent care should it be required needs to be factored into the treatment plan. Should a child require general anesthesia, a conservative pulpal procedure (eg, direct pulp capping, partial pulpotomy), which would be considered for a patient requiring less behavior guidance, may not be performed. When a patient is treated under general anesthesia, the clinician may consider a more aggressive treatment, such as full pulpotomy or pulpectomy, because of the inability to assess the

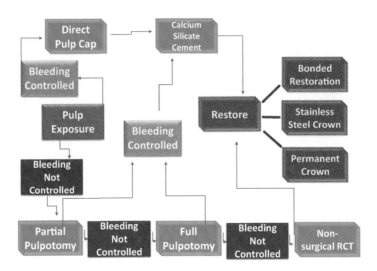

Fig. 1. A decision tree on how to manage young pulp exposures in the adolescent permanent dentition. RCT, root canal treatment.

health of the remaining pulp tissue. Clinicians must always consider what the action plan will be should emergent care needs arise.

Classically, the objective of endodontic therapy has been the prevention and/or treatment of apical periodontitis. The diagnosis of reversible or irreversible pulpitis is controversial in relation to the state of the pulp because of the absence of noninvasive techniques for determining the severity of pulp inflammation.[30] Furthermore, current material science has now provided predictable therapies to manage the dental pulp. Increased awareness and education of clinicians on how to optimally manage the pulp tissue should be of the utmost priority.[8]

Vital Pulp Therapies

The European Society of Endodontology's position statement on the management of deep caries and exposed pulp defines vital pulp therapy as strategies designed to maintain the health of all or part of the pulp[31] (**Box 1**). The development of calcium silicate cements (eg, Pro-Root MTA, BC putty, Bio-Dentine) over the past 2 decades has permitted predictable vital pulp therapies to be performed with success and survivability well into the 90% range.[32–36]

The current American Association of Endodontists diagnostic terminology designates pulpitis into reversible and irreversible pulpitis.[6] The direct assessment of the pulp tissue, ideally using a surgical microscope, must direct the decision on how much pulp will need to be removed to reach healthy uninflamed tissue and whether a vital pulp therapy will be attempted.[6,23]

Direct pulp capping

When an exposure of the dental pulp occurs from either a carious or mechanical cause, a direct pulp cap may be considered based on the clinical observation and control of the bleeding from the exposed pulp tissues.[37] Hemorrhage controlled with gentle pressure applied with a cotton pellet soaked with full-strength 5.25% sodium hypochlorite for several minutes (up to 5 minutes) may be considered for direct pulp cap. Other factors also need to be considered, such as the size of the exposure.

Box 1
Vital pulp treatment definitions and terminology/glossary published by the European Society of Endodontology

Direct pulp capping
  Following the preservation of an aseptic working field, application of a biomaterial directly onto the exposed pulp, before immediate placement of a permanent restoration.
    Class I
      No preoperative presence of a deep carious lesion. Pulp exposure judged clinically to be through sound dentine with an expectation that the underlying pulp tissue is healthy (exposure caused by a traumatic injury to the tooth or an iatrogenic exposure).
    Class II
      Preoperative presence of a deep or extremely deep carious lesion. Pulp exposure judged clinically to be through a zone of bacterial contamination with an expectation that the underlying pulp tissue is inflamed. Enhanced operative protocol recommended (aseptic procedure using magnification, disinfectant, and application of a hydraulic calcium silicate cement).

Partial pulpotomy
  Removal of a small portion of coronal pulp tissue after exposure, followed by application of a biomaterial directly onto the remaining pulp tissue before placement of a permanent restoration.

Full pulpotomy
  Complete removal of the coronal pulp and application of a biomaterial directly onto the pulp tissue at the level of the root canal orifices, before placement of a permanent restoration.

From Duncan HF, Galler KM, Tomson PL, et al. European Society of Endodontology position statement: Management of deep caries and the exposed pulp. Int Endod J 2019;52(7):923-34.

Studies have shown that exposures up to 2.5 mm have very high success following the use of current calcium silicate cements. Exposures greater than 2.5 mm may be better candidates for partial or full pulpotomy.[38] Consideration also must be given to the general dental status of the adolescent patient, and the likelihood that little may change in the patient's home care and dietary habits that led to the current dental condition. Clinicians must consider whether the dental pulp has a stronger likelihood of avoiding future disorder if more restorative material can be placed between the pulp and the oral cavity as permitted by pulpotomy.

A summary of the direct pulp capping technique is available in **Box 2** and **Fig. 2**.

Box 2
Summary of technique for direct pulp capping treatment

1. Rubber dam isolation/disinfection of the suspected tooth

2. Complete caries excavation working from the peripheral margin inward to the deepest caries; caries indicator dye is recommended

3. Assessment of the size of the exposure (<2.5 mm)

4. Placement of a cotton pellet soaked with full-strength 5.25% sodium hypochlorite for up to 5 minutes

5. Assessment of bleeding from the site

6. Placement of a 2-mm thickness of the calcium silicate cement directly over the exposed pulp

7. Immediate restoration of the tooth

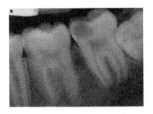 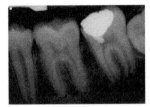 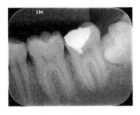

Preoperative   Postoperative   3-year follow-up

Fig. 2. Direct pulp capping treatment after carious exposure. A direct pulp capping was performed, removing all carious and infected dentin and inflamed pulp tissue from the pulp horn. Healthy uninflamed pulp tissue was treated with calcium silicate cement followed by permanent restoration.

Partial/full pulpotomy

The decision to proceed with pulpotomy (partial or full) has several subjective and extrinsic factors at play in the decision. The clinical determination that the pulp amputation has reached the level of uninflamed pulp tissue is the first and most critical decision.[6] The ability to provide immediate emergent care should the conservative procedure not work also needs to be considered. The influence of a third-party insurance provider could affect a parent's acceptance of treatment as well as approval for the future restoration. These extrinsic factors can be among the biggest obstacles to providing a predictable, biologically sound procedure.[1] Clinicians need to be ready to explain the benefits of conservatively maintaining the vital tissue for continued root development both apically and along the canal wall (ie, the presence of a vital tissue to maintain the intrapulpal pressure/outward flow of dentinal fluid through the tubules, and a vital tissue to mount an immunologic response to future bacterial invasion). These biological benefits also provide an intrinsic native barrier for the health of the periapical tissues.[39]

Once it has been determined that a pulpotomy will be attempted and a current diagnosis of the dental pulp has been made, the procedure begins as with any other procedure that involves dental pulp management, with proper rubber dam isolation and disinfection of the tooth with a 0.12% chlorhexidine scrub. The carious lesion is excavated from the peripheral margins inward toward the site of exposure. Once the pulp has been exposed, the clinician should change to a diamond bur on a high-speed handpiece with copious water irrigation to amputate the dental pulp to the level of healthy pulp tissue. This process may result in a portion of the coronal pulp tissue remaining (partial pulpotomy) or carried to the canal orifices or into the canals to reach healthy tissue if needed. The partial pulpotomy has the advantage of maintaining the cell-rich coronal pulp tissue over the less cellular cervical pulp tissue in the full pulpotomy.[4,40]

The authors do not recommend performing pulp amputation with a carbide bur because the risk of tearing and removing healthy tissues from the root canal system is very high. At this point, visual assessment of the pulp and assessment of hemorrhage following the placement of a 5.25% sodium hypochlorite cotton pellet for up to 5 minutes is performed. If bleeding is not controlled, the pulp amputation needs to be carried deeper into the inflamed canal or a change in treatment to a pulpectomy must be considered. Once noninflamed pulp tissue is reached, the placement of 2 mm of a calcium silicate cement material covering the exposed pulp tissue followed by a permanent restoration is recommended.

Box 3
Summary of technique for partial/full pulpotomy treatment

1. Isolation/disinfection of the tooth
2. Caries removal with a carbide bur; caries indicator dye recommended
3. Exposure of the pulp and change to a diamond bur
4. Removal of the pulp to the level of visually healthy pulp tissue
5. Hemorrhage control with a cotton pellet soaked with full-strength 5.25% sodium hypochlorite for up to 5 minutes
6. Placement of 2 mm of calcium silicate cement
7. Permanent restoration

A summary of the partial/full pulpotomy technique is available in **Box 3** and **Fig. 3**.

Pulpectomy/Nonsurgical Endodontic Therapy/Revascularization

Nonsurgical endodontic therapy (pulpectomy) technically is no different than that performed on adult patients. The decision that may need to be addressed is how to manage a tooth with an open apex. Historically, this was done using long-term calcium hydroxide for apexification or apexogenesis. Andreasen and colleagues[41] showed that the use of calcium hydroxide beyond 30 days caused a weakening of the dentin that led to an increased chance of tooth fracture. The placement of a calcium silicate cement apical plug has replaced the long-term calcium hydroxide treatment and allows immediate obturation of the canals. Placement of the apical plug can be a challenging technique. A large gutta-percha cone approximating the canal diameter can be used to initiate condensation of the calcium silicate cement material. The cone should be fitted 2 to 3 mm short of the apical foramen. The material is carried into the canal and condensed with the gutta-percha cone into the apical third of the tooth.

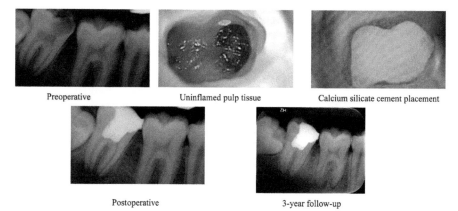

Preoperative   Uninflamed pulp tissue   Calcium silicate cement placement

Postoperative   3-year follow-up

Fig. 3. Full pulpotomy treatment after carious exposure. A full pulpotomy was performed, removing all carious and infected dentin and inflamed pulp tissue at the level of the root canal orifices. Healthy uninflamed pulp tissue was treated with calcium silicate cement followed by permanent restoration.

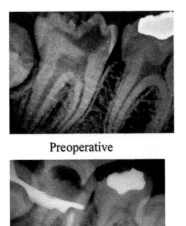
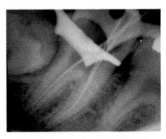

Preoperative   Complete instrumentation

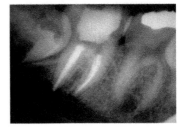

Conventional obturation of the mesial roots and   Complete obturation
calcium silicate cement plug on the distal root

Fig. 4. Pulpectomy with calcium silicate cement plug of tooth with irreversible pulpitis. A pulpectomy was performed, removing all inflamed pulp tissue. Mesial roots were conventionally obturated with gutta-percha and a calcium silicate cement plug was placed to seal the open apex of the underdeveloped distal root followed by conventional canal obturation and permanent restoration.

The condensation needs to be radiographically confirmed before backfilling with gutta-percha (**Fig. 4**). Once the decision to place an apical plug has been made, most follow-up treatments, if necessary, would require apical surgery or extraction. For this reason, the authors recommend that, in root canals where an apical stop and gutta-percha obturation can be achieved, gutta-percha obturation is still the preferred method.

Revascularization has become a predictable and successful procedure for the undeveloped root of the necrotic dental pulp[11–13,27,42] (**Fig. 5**).

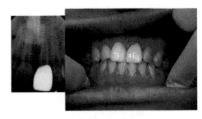

Preoperative   Postoperative   9-year follow-up   10-year follow-up

Fig. 5. Revascularization treatment after trauma. An 8-year-old child presented with an immature necrotic permanent maxillary central incisor as a result of trauma. Following the 2011 American Association of Endodontics' protocol at that time, revascularization was performed followed by conservative restoration. Permanent restoration was placed after the completion of growth and development of the patient.

SUMMARY

1. The continued development of better dental materials and the resiliency of the dental pulp in adolescent patients have expanded the treatment options available currently.
2. Pulp therapy modalities include management of the vital dental pulp, immediate management of the open apex during traditional endodontic treatment, and current expansion of revascularization/regeneration techniques to provide the ingrowth of new pulplike tissues into the root canal space.
3. The decade-long success of revascularization procedures in children has spurred great interest in developing methods of regenerating part, if not all, of the dental pulp.
4. Several researchers have already performed in vivo studies investigating various cell-based and cell-homing methods of pulp regeneration.
5. Future development of a shelf-stable ready-to-use material to regenerate a new pulplike tissue in teeth of adolescent patients is awaited.

CLINICS CARE POINTS

- Vital pulp tissue provides continued root development and an immunologic barrier to protect the periapical tissue.
- Pulp vitality testing is not the determinant for the degree of pulp damage.
- Disinfection and proper rubber dam isolation are essential.
- A definitive treatment option is based on visual examination of the exposed pulp.
- Diamond burs, run on water-cooled high-speed handpieces, are used to amputate all pulp tissues.
- Hemostatic agents are never used for the control of pulpal hemorrhage.
- A minimum of 2 mm of calcium silicate cement should cover all exposed pulp tissue.
- A definitive restoration should be placed immediately after vital pulp therapy.

DISCLOSURE

The authors have nothing to disclose.

REFERENCES

1. Al-Madi EM, Al Saleh SA, Bukhary SM, et al. Endodontic and restorative treatment patterns of pulpally involved immature permanent posterior teeth. Int J Dent 2018;1–5. https://doi.org/10.1155/2018/2178535.
2. Slutzky-Goldberg I, Slutzky H, Gorfil C, et al. Restoration of endodontically treated teeth review and treatment recommendations. Int J Dent 2009;2009. https://doi.org/10.1155/2009/150251.
3. Ray HA, Trope M. Periapical status of endodontically treated teeth in relation to the technical quality of the root filling and the coronal restoration. Int Endod J 1995;28(1):12–8.
4. Chailertvanitkul P, Paphangkorakit J, Sooksantisakoonchai N, et al. Randomized control trial comparing calcium hydroxide and mineral trioxide aggregate for partial pulpotomies in cariously exposed pulps of permanent molars. Int Endod J 2014;47(9):835–42.

5. American Academy of Pediatric Dentistry. Pulp therapy for primary and immature permanent teeth. The Reference Manual of Pediatric Dentistry. Chicago (IL): American Academy of Pediatric Dentistry; 2020. p. 384–92.

6. American Association of Endodontists Position Statement on Vital Pulp Therapy. 2021. Available at: https://www.aae.org/specialty/clinical-resources/guidelines-position-statements/. Accessed April 30, 2021.

7. Bjørndal L, Demant S, Dabelsteen S. Depth and activity of carious lesions as indicators for the regenerative potential of dental pulp after intervention. J Endod 2014;40(4 Suppl):S76–81.

8. Bjørndal L, Simon S, Tomson PL, et al. Management of deep caries and the exposed pulp. Int Endod J 2019;52(7):949–73.

9. Casagrande L, Cordeiro MM, Nör SA, et al. Dental pulp stem cells in regenerative dentistry. Odontology 2011;99(1):1–7.

10. Ravindran S, Huang CC, George A. Extracellular matrix of dental pulp stem cells: applications in pulp tissue engineering using somatic MSCs. Front Physiol 2014; 4:395.

11. Hargreaves KM, Giesler T, Henry M, et al. Regeneration potential of the young permanent tooth: what does the future hold? Pediatr Dent 2008;30(3):253–60.

12. Trope M. Regenerative potential of dental pulp. J Endod 2008;34(7 Suppl):S13–7.

13. Nor JE, Cucco C. The future: Stem cells and biological approaches for pulp regeneration. In: Fuks A, Peretz B, editors. Pediatric endodontics current concepts in pulp therapy for primary and young permanent teeth. New York: Springer; 2016. p. 149–61.

14. Kawashima N, Okiji T. Odontoblasts: Specialized hard-tissue-forming cells in the dentin-pulp complex. Congenit Anom 2016;56(4):144–53.

15. Byers MR, Taylor PE, Khayat BG, et al. Effects of injury and inflammation on pulpal and periapical nerves. J Endod 1990;16(2):78–84.

16. Hargreaves KM, Bowles WR, Jackson DL. Intrinsic regulation of CGRP release by dental pulp sympathetic fibers. J Dent Res 2003;82(5):398–401.

17. Kim S. Neurovascular interactions in the dental pulp in health and inflammation. J Endod 1990;16(2):48–53.

18. Tønder KJ. Vascular reactions in the dental pulp during inflammation. Acta Odontol Scand 1983;41(4):247–56.

19. Takahashi K. Changes in the pulpal vasculature during inflammation. J Endod 1990;16(2):92–7.

20. Seltzer S, Bender IB, Ziontz M. The dynamics of pulp inflammation: correlations between diagnostic data and actual histologic findings in the pulp. Oral Surg Oral Med Oral Pathol 1963;16:846–71.

21. Dummer PM, Hicks R, Huws D. Clinical signs and symptoms in pulp disease. Int Endod J 1980;13(1):27–35.

22. Ricucci D, Loghin S, Siqueira JF Jr. Correlation between clinical and histologic pulp diagnoses. J Endod 2014;40(12):1932–9.

23. Ricucci D, Siqueira JF Jr, Li Y, et al. Vital pulp therapy: histopathology and histobacteriology-based guidelines to treat teeth with deep caries and pulp exposure. J Dent 2019;86:41–52.

24. Bender IB. Reversible and irreversible painful pulpitides: Diagnosis and treatment. Aust Endod J 2000;26(1):10–4.

25. Camp JH. Diagnosis dilemmas in vital pulp therapy: Treatment for the toothache is changing, especially in young, immature teeth. Pediatr Dent 2008;30(3): 197–205.

26. Zanini M, Meyer E, Simon S. Pulp Inflammation Diagnosis from Clinical to Inflammatory Mediators: A Systematic Review. J Endod 2017;43(7):1033–51.
27. Nuni E. Pulp therapy for the young permanent dentition. In: Fuks A, Peretz B, editors. Pediatric endodontics current concepts in pulp therapy for primary and young permanent teeth. New York: Springer; 2016. p. 117–48.
28. Abu-Tahun I, Torabinejad M. Management of teeth with vital pulps and open apices. Endod Top 2012;23:79–104.
29. St Paul A, Phillips C, Lee JY, et al. Provider perceptions of treatment options for immature permanent teeth. J Endod 2017;43(6):910–5.
30. Bjørndal L. The caries process and its effect on the pulp: the science is changing and so is our understanding. J Endod 2008;34(7 Suppl):S2–5.
31. Duncan HF, Galler KM, Tomson PL, et al. European Society of Endodontology position statement: Management of deep caries and the exposed pulp. Int Endod J 2019;52(7):923–34.
32. Witherspoon DE. Vital pulp therapy with new materials: new directions and treatment perspectives-permanent teeth. Pediatr Dent 2008;30(3):220–4.
33. Aguilar P, Linsuwanont P. Vital pulp therapy in vital permanent teeth with cariously exposed pulp: a systematic review. J Endod 2011;37(5):581–7.
34. Utneja S, Nawal RR, Talwar S, et al. Current perspectives of bio-ceramic technology in endodontics: calcium enriched mixture cement - review of its composition, properties and applications. Restor Dent Endod 2015;40(1):1–13.
35. Awawdeh L, Al-Qudah A, Hamouri H, et al. Outcomes of Vital Pulp Therapy Using Mineral Trioxide Aggregate or Biodentine: A Prospective Randomized Clinical Trial. J Endod 2018;44(11):1603–9.
36. Suhag K, Duhan J, Tewari S, et al. Success of Direct Pulp Capping Using Mineral Trioxide Aggregate and Calcium Hydroxide in Mature Permanent Molars with Pulps Exposed during Carious Tissue Removal: 1-year Follow-up. J Endod 2019;45(7):840–7.
37. Bogen G, Kim JS, Bakland LK. Direct pulp capping with mineral trioxide aggregate: an observational study. J Am Dent Assoc 2008;139(3):305–15.
38. Edwards D, Stone S, Bailey O, et al. Preserving pulp vitality: part two - vital pulp therapies. Br Dent J 2021;230(3):148–55.
39. Hahn CL, Liewehr FR. Innate immune responses of the dental pulp to caries. J Endod 2007;33(6):643–51.
40. Elmsmari F, Ruiz XF, Miró Q, et al. Outcome of partial pulpotomy in cariously exposed posterior permanent teeth: A Systematic Review and Meta-analysis. J Endod 2019;45(11):1296–306.e3.
41. Andreasen JO, Farik B, Munksgaard EC. Long-term calcium hydroxide as a root canal dressing may increase risk of root fracture. Dent Traumatol 2002;18(3):134–7.
42. Banchs F, Trope M. Revascularization of immature permanent teeth with apical periodontitis: new treatment protocol? J Endod 2004;30(4):196–200.

Adolescent Orofacial Trauma

Mark Sosovicka, DMD[a],*, Matthew DeMerle, DDS, MD[b]

KEYWORDS

- Adolescent facial fractures • Soft tissue injuries • Lacerations
- Traumatic dental injuries • Dentoalveolar fractures

KEY POINTS

- Adolescent facial traumatic soft tissue injuries and traumatic dental injuries are commom and facial fractures although uncommon may be associated with other significant injuries including neurological injuries.
- Initial management of pediatric facial trauma involves stabilizing the patient from a physiologic standpoint before evaluation or imaging of the facial injuries.
- Adolescent facial fractures are often "greenstick" with minimal displacement and may be treated conservatively with observation, while displaced mandible fractures with malocclusion are treated by reestablishing the occlusion with maxillomandibular fixation.
- Soft tissue lacerations are evaluated for underlying injuries and repaired following irrigation and debridement.
- Traumatic dental injuries, including tooth avulsion, should be treated promptly with the goal of maintaining the tooth with early replantation and splinting with periodic reevaluation for possble endodontic therapy.

ADOLESCENT FACIAL TRAUMA

Trauma affects hundreds of thousands of patients and costs billions of dollars annually in the United States. The pediatric population is a subset that deserves special attention due to multiple factors, including but not limited to anatomy, mechanism of injury, future growth considerations, sex, and age. Despite craniofacial trauma being frequent in pediatric patients, the most common injuries are usually soft tissue and dentoalveolar injuries. Facial fractures in children are relatively infrequent versus adults, but may be associated with severe injuries and significant morbidity and associated disability. Important goals of management of facial trauma in pediatric patients is focused on initially stabilizing the patient, identifying any other concomitant severe injuries, and then diagnosis and management of the facial injuries.[1]

[a] Department of Oral and Maxillofacial Surgery, University of Pittsburgh School of Dental Medicine, 3501 Terrace Street, Pittsburgh, PA 15261, USA; [b] Department of Oral and Maxillofacial Surgery, University of Pittsburgh Medical Center, 200 Lothrop Street, Pittsburgh, PA 15213, USA
* Corresponding author.
E-mail address: sosovickam@upmc.edu

Dent Clin N Am 65 (2021) 787–804
https://doi.org/10.1016/j.cden.2021.07.005
0011-8532/21/© 2021 Elsevier Inc. All rights reserved.

dental.theclinics.com

OROFACIAL TRAUMA DEMOGRAPHICS

A review of the National Trauma Data Bank of 2016 from the American College of Surgeons gives an overall view of pediatric trauma, highlighting differences in trauma prevalence as follows.[2] Trauma is the leading cause of morbidity and mortality in children, with the head being the most frequently involved and the face the fourth most common affected anatomic region at 24.3% of all cases. Rates of pediatric trauma vary by age, with a mild increase in incidence at the 5 to 7 age range (~6000 cases) and again at 11 to 18 years of age (~5000 up to 12,000 cases per year by age 18). These increases can likely be attributed to the increased activity in school-age children 5 to 7 years old and again with ever-increasing levels of activity in pre-teens and teenage patients. There is also a difference by sex, with boys showing a 1.35 to 1.5 times higher incidence of trauma than girls in the 1-year to 9-year age groups. However, male incidence continues to increase during adolescence (ages 11–18) whereas female trauma somewhat levels off. Incidence also can be categorized by intent, with unintentional injury being an overwhelming majority at 88.2% of all pediatric trauma, although potential child abuse must always be considered.

ANATOMY

Pediatric craniofacial anatomy must be given special consideration, as the skeletal anatomy changes with growth and development of the child through adolescence. The pediatric facial skeleton has incomplete ossification and compliant suture lines, making it more flexible than the adult facial skeleton. Children also have a larger cranial body-to-mass ratio than adults, and the malar region is protected by a relatively larger malar fat pad. These differences result in a unique distribution of facial injuries in the pediatric population. With the larger cranial size, fractures of the skull vault are more commonly seen in children. Maxillary and midface fractures are also more common in younger children, whereas mandible fractures are more commonly seen in adolescents and adults. Pediatric patients also have a lower incidence of severely displaced facial fractures, as increased skeletal flexibility often resulting in "greenstick" nondisplaced fractures of the face.

PATIENT EVALUATION

Pediatric patients with facial trauma must first be stabilized by Advanced Trauma Life Support protocol with an emphasis on detection and treatment of life-threatening injuries.[3] Pediatric patients have a higher risk for physiologic decompensation due to increased body surface area to blood volume ratios, low blood volume, and higher cardiac output with increased metabolic rate and oxygen demands. Resultant hemodynamic instability makes pediatric patients prone to hypotension, hypoxia, and hypothermia secondary to traumatic injuries. As with any trauma patient, care should be taken to perform an overall assessment of the patient before evaluation of specific facial injuries. Injuries that may require acute intervention may go unnoticed if the provider does not follow the correct sequence of the *ABCDEs* of acute pediatric trauma evaluation in the following discussion.

A. *Airway* assessment and possible establishment of a patent airway. Pediatric airway obstruction is common due to a large flaccid tongue and pharyngeal soft tissue, and possible intraoral hemorrhage or foreign body obstruction. Airway evaluation and treatment, including possible airway repositioning with head tilt chin lift or jaw thrust or use of airway adjuncts such as oral or nasopharyngeal airways, or possible intubation, may be required. Airway evaluation and its management are the first priorities, as pediatric trauma–related airway compromise and respiratory arrest are the most common causes of cardiac arrest in pediatric patients.

B. *Breathing* with the ability to ventilate the lungs for oxygenation of blood and removal of carbon dioxide. Pediatric respiratory rates decrease with age, with infants having a rate of 30 to 40 times per minute to 15 to 20 times per minute in teenagers. Lung tidal volume also increases from 4 to 6 mL in infants to 6 to 8 mL/kg in adolescents.

C. *Circulation and control of bleeding.* Pediatric craniofacial injuries can result in significant blood loss. Vital signs should be closely monitored for signs of hemodynamic instability and any large bleeding vessels should be controlled with hemostats or gauze pressure. Pediatric patients may often tolerate a loss of up to one-third of total blood volume before developing hypotension due to compensation with tachycardia to maintain systolic blood pressure.

D. *Disability* from pediatric head injuries may result, including central nervous system injuries, such as traumatic brain injuries or concussions. Use of the Glasgow Coma Scale (**Table 1**) with motor, eye-opening, and verbal responses are evaluated and correlated with head injury severity and possible need for immediate treatment, including possible cervical spine immobilization. Concussions are commonly associated with pediatric facial trauma and defined as altered mental status with or without loss of consciousness. Most post–concussion-related symptoms resolve within 3 months and there is no specific directed therapy for concussions.

E. *Exposure* of the injured with completely undressing and examining the child or adolescent for a full trauma assessment to rule out other injuries while preventing hypothermia of the patient. A fast and reliable method to assess the *ABCDE*s in age-appropriate pediatric patients is to ask the patient their name and what happened. If the patient is able to verbally respond, this suggests the airway is not compromised, and the patient can breathe well enough for speech production.

Table 1 Glasgow coma scale		
Response	**Scale**	**Score**
Eye-opening response	Eyes open spontaneously	4 Points
	Eyes open to verbal command, speech, or shout	3 Points
	Eyes open to pain (not applied to face)	2 Points
	No eye opening	1 Point
Verbal response	Oriented	5 Points
	Confused conversation, but able to answer questions	4 Points
	Inappropriate responses, words discernible	3 Points
	Incomprehensible sounds or speech	2 Points
	No verbal response	1 Point
Motor response	Obeys commands for movement	6 Points
	Purposeful movement to painful stimulus	5 Points
	Withdraws from pain	4 Points
	Abnormal (spastic) flexion, decorticate posture	3 Points
	Extensor (rigid) response, decerebrate posture	2 Points
	No motor response	1 Point

Minor brain injury = 13 to 15 points; moderate brain injury = 9 to 12 points; severe brain injury = 3 to 8 points.

If the patient is conscious and alert enough to describe what happened, this indicates generalized neurologic stability. Vital signs are continually assessed to ensure adequate cardiac and respiratory function. Failure to respond to these questions in an age-appropriate manner or abnormalities of any vital signs indicate compromised physiologic stability and may warrant acute management.

Once the primary survey has been completed (assessment of the *ABCDE*s) and the patient is stable, then the secondary survey can begin. The secondary survey is a complete head-to-toe assessment of the patient, which includes physical examination of all body areas and patient history, while continually reassessing vital signs. During this time, a complete neurologic examination is completed and imaging is obtained to rule out any suspected head or neck injuries.

DIAGNOSTIC IMAGING

Radiographic imaging should be obtained in most acute trauma cases, unless there are extenuating circumstances that would preclude the patient from having these images taken. Also, in the case of isolated soft tissue injuries secondary to low-impact trauma, imaging is not indicated if the examination is otherwise normal. However, there should be a low threshold for obtaining imaging if there is any suspicion of possible facial fractures or possible foreign bodies in the wound.

PANORAMIC TOMOGRAPHY

In many cases, the most readily available imaging for the practicing dentist will be a panoramic radiograph. This can be useful when the trauma is limited to the mandible and lower midface; however, it will have limited utility when evaluating other regions of the upper facial skeleton. The use of the panoramic radiograph still has some utility, especially for evaluation of the dentition and dentoalveolar fractures.

COMPUTED TOMOGRAPHY

Computed tomography (CT) imaging with 1-mm to 4-mm slices has multiple advantages over panoramic radiographs, including multiple planes of image, avoidance of superimposed structures, and larger field of view. Axial slice thickness of 1 mm is useful for greater image fidelity as well as reformatting for possible 3-dimensional reconstruction. The use of CT imaging does expose pediatric patients to an increased level of radiation of approximately 1 to 10 millisieverts (mSv), compared with the average person exposed to 3 mSv due to natural ionizing radiation yearly.[4] CT imaging should enhance information from a thorough clinical examination. The increased radiation dose in pediatric patients must be considered, as pediatric patients are more sensitive to radiation than adults, have a longer life expectancy than adults, and increased radiation risk for possible development of brain tumors or leukemia.[5]

HEAD AND NECK EXAMINATION

When evaluating a patient with facial trauma, it is helpful for the provider to have a standardized examination to assess the face by regions, including the cranium/skull base, frontal region, orbits, nose/nasal bones, temporomandibular joint/ears, maxilla and mandible, and intraoral examination.

Starting with the *cranium*, evaluate for any lacerations, contusions, or obvious fractures. This should include visual examination and digital palpation for palpable defects or depressions. The retro-auricular/mastoid region is assessed for "Battle's sign" hematoma of mastoid areas of the skull behind the ears associated with skull base fractures. Cranial scalp lacerations may lead to significant blood loss and should be promptly treated.

Attention can then be turned to the *frontal* region, looking again for any irregularities, including skull defects, depression, or crepitus. Frontal sinus fractures may require treatment if depressed or if there is involvement of the posterior table with possible dural tears and cerebrospinal fluid leak through the nose. Also, V1 trigeminal nerve branch paresthesia/numbness of the forehead region may be present. These findings sometimes can be masked in the acute phase by swelling, so axial CT images are helpful in assessing the anterior and posterior tables of the frontal sinus and nasofrontal outflow tract.

Examination of the *orbits* then would follow with evaluation for ecchymosis and edema of the periorbital region as well as orbital trauma such as subconjunctival (scleral) hemorrhage or enophthalmos (sunken in eye appearance). Vision defects due to cranial nerve II (optic) and/or extraocular movement defects with cranial nerves III (oculomotor), IV (trochlear), or VI (abducens) involvement resulting in limited eye gaze or diplopia (double vision) require an ophthalmology consultation. Orbital floor "blow-out" fractures are common in pediatric facial trauma patients as a protective mechanism to prevent injury to the eye. Orbital floor fractures may result in limited upward eye gaze due to inferior rectus muscle entrapment of the affected eye resulting in diplopia. Orbital floor fractures with entrapment require inferior rectus muscle release within 48 hours to prevent muscle atrophy or fibrosis and repair of the orbital floor fracture with an implant via a transconjunctival inner eyelid incision.[6]

The *nasal* region examination can be concurrent with orbital examination. The external nose is inspected for gross deviation from the facial midline or bony steps or crepitus of the thin nasal bones or nasal septum. As previously discussed, nasal bone or nasal septal fractures are a common pediatric facial fracture with possible functional and nasal airflow, deviation, or cosmetic defects, which are anatomically reduced by closed reduction with possible internal and/or external nasal splinting. Evaluation for naso-orbital ethmoidal (NOE) fractures should be performed and may result in traumatic telecanthus (increased intercanthal width of the eyes) and widened and flattening of the superior nasal bridge area. Axial view on CT imaging will be helpful in evaluation of the degree of displacement and comminution of the fractures. Any nasal septal hematomas should be evacuated to prevent possible necrosis of the septal cartilage and loss of nasal support. Significant NOE fractures are treated with open reduction with rigid internal fixation with miniplates and screws or transnasal wiring to prevent traumatic telecanthus and widening of the upper nose.

Maxillary assessment begins during the orbital examination, looking for any fractures by palpation for step defect depressions of the inferior orbital rim. The malar and zygomatic regions should also be examined visually and palpated for fractures and depressions that may not be detected on physical examination due to acute swelling. Some zygomaticomaxillary (ZMC) fractures can impinge on the mandibular coronoid process, resulting in trismus (limited mandibular opening), flattening of the malar eminence or cheek, and may result in a unilateral trigeminal nerve V2 branch paresthesia of the upper teeth and lip, lateral nose, and cheek. Nondisplaced fractures of the zygomatic arch or ZMC may be observed with the patient to maintain a soft diet and avoiding any contact or trauma to the face or head for 6 to 8 weeks. LeFort fractures can cause mobility of the maxilla, nasal, and zygomatic areas, which can be tested by grasping the maxilla bilaterally apical to the anterior teeth and checking for maxillary mobility. A mobile dentoalveolar fracture involving multiple tooth segments may be present with fracture of the alveolar bone and associated teeth and require stabilization with bonded splinting of the teeth or possible open miniplate fixation.

MANDIBLE

The mandible should be examined with palpation for step defects of the inferior border, crepitus of bone with palpation, malocclusion with open bite, premature contacts or posterior edge-to-edge cusp occlusion, trismus, deviation of the mandibular dental midline with opening, mandibular gingival tears, and vestibular or floor of the mouth ecchymosis. The mandibular examination should include a thorough temporomandibular joint (TMJ) examination to evaluate for TMJ pain, clicking, crepitus, dysfunction, or trismus possibly associated with mandibular condylar process or subcondylar fractures. Condylar process or subcondylar fractures may result in deviation to the side of the fracture due to associated loss of posterior vertical dimension on the side of the fracture. If the mandible fracture involves the inferior alveolar canal with displacement of the fracture, the patient may have a V3 paresthesia (altered sensation of numbness or tingling) of the lower lip on the side of the fracture.

Previously the panoramic radiograph was the standard for evaluation of mandible fractures often due to availability, although often CT imaging is obtained in the hospital and provides 3-dimensional images of mandible fractures. The vector of force to the mandible may result in specific fracture patterns. For example, if a patient is struck on the left body of the mandible, the resultant fracture pattern is often a left-sided angle, body, or parasymphyseal fracture with a contralateral condylar process or subcondylar fracture. Another example would be a fall in which the patient strikes their chin on the ground, which can often result in bilateral condylar process or subcondylar fractures.

The *ear* should be examined for hematoma formation and laceration. Any hematomas of the ears should be evacuated to prevent necrosis of the underlying ear cartilage and lacerations are repaired with sutures and covered with a pressure dressing to prevent hematoma formation. Care also should be taken to look for the presence of exudate from the external auditory canal, including blood or clear fluid, which may indicate a cerebrospinal fluid leak. A gross hearing test for each ear to evaluate cranial nerve VIII (vestibulocochlear) and tympanic membrane function should be completed.

MANDIBULAR FRACTURE TREATMENT

When considering treatment of facial fractures, one must consider the type, location, and severity of the fracture. There are also multiple patient-based factors, including patient age, activity level, and compliance to proposed treatment. Some mandibular fractures in the adult population may warrant open reduction with internal rigid plate and screw fixation, whereas the same fractures in the pediatric population may require conservative treatment with observation, a soft non-chew diet, or maintenance of occlusion by closed reduction techniques, as discussed next.

MANDIBULAR CLOSED REDUCTION METHODS

Closed reduction of mandibular fractures with maxillomandibular fixation (MMF) or intermaxillary fixation (IMF) are used interchangeably and may be completed by several common methods to establish and maintain the pretrauma dental occlusion. In certain cases, closed reduction with MMF or IMF may be the only treatment required for many mandibular fractures. A variety of closed reduction techniques may be used and can be performed in either an inpatient or outpatient setting, under local anesthesia or with sedation or general anesthesia if needed. Care should be taken to not disturb the developing tooth buds of the permanent dentition while treating pediatric mandibular fractures. MMF or IMF are techniques that avoid trauma to the developing tooth buds and may require circummandibular symphysis wire and a piriform nasal aperture wire for attachment. Then they are connected with a fixation wire for MMF or IMF.

Ivy loop fixation uses stainless steel wires around 2 adjacent teeth in each quadrant using circumdental 24-gauge wires with a buccal wire loop. A 24-gauge fixation wire is then passed through both the maxillary and mandibular loop and tightened to place the patient in MMF. This is a simple, low-cost, effective treatment, especially for pediatric patients who are easy to place under local or possible deep sedation/general anesthesia. The image in **Fig. 1** demonstrates placement and configuration of Ivy loops.

Arch bar fixation also uses the patient's occlusion for fracture reduction, and Erich arch bars are routinely placed on the maxillary and mandibular teeth for means of MMF and use 24-gauge stainless steel circumdental wires that are passed around each individual tooth below the cingulum or height of contour and then wrapped around the arch bar. The patient then is placed into their habitual centric occlusion and fixation wires are passed around the lugs of the maxillary and mandibular arch bars, tightened, and twisted in a "rosette" to complete the MMF, as demonstrated in **Fig. 2**. The arch bars may also be used with orthodontic elastics for traction to guide the patient's bite and occlusion by nonrigid fixation once the wire fixation is removed. Elastic fixation also is used to permit TMJ movement and prevent possible TMJ dysfunction or TMJ ankylosis in pediatric patients with condylar head or intracapsular fractures with prolonged rigid wire fixation.

Intermaxillary fixation screws (IMF screws) also may be used to perform closed mandibular reductions with MMF. The closed reduction is completed with the use of IMF screws placed into the alveolar bone of the maxilla and mandibular quadrants apical to the tooth roots. Fixation wires are then passed from the maxillary to mandibular screws, as seen in the image (**Fig. 3**).

Care must be taken with the pediatric trauma population to avoid trauma to developing permanent tooth buds if IMF screws are used. The use of IMF screws and wires

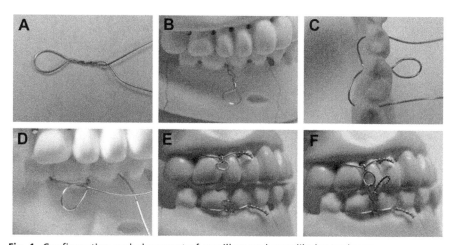

Fig. 1. Configuration and placement of maxillary and mandibular Ivy loops.

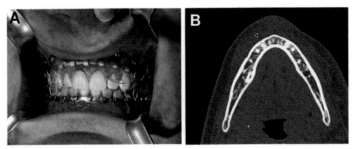

Fig. 2. (*A, B*) Arch bar maxillomandibular fixation and cone-beam CT of patient's mandible with fracture noted by dotted arrow.

is generally quick and easy to place. Following closed reduction of mandibular fractures by the preceding techniques, malocclusions are rare and dental compensation will restore a normal occlusion.

OPEN REDUCTION AND RIGID INTERNAL FIXATION

Open reduction and rigid internal fixation (ORIF) may be used in cases in which a mandible fracture is not amenable to closed treatment due to severe displacement, comminuted fractures, or a compromised occlusion that limits closed reduction. ORIF involves a surgical procedure in which the fractures are opened with intraoral or extraoral incisions, anatomically "reduced" or realigned, and rigidly fixated with titanium low-profile plates and screws. If rigid plate and screw fixation is used for maxillary or mandibular fractures in the pediatric population, again trauma to permanent tooth buds or immature apices of teeth should be avoided. The use of fixation plates

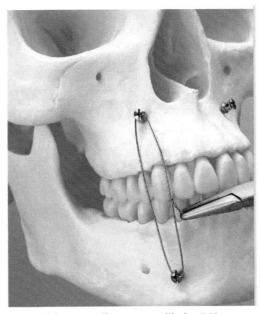

Fig. 3. Fixation wires passed from maxillary to mandibular IMF screws.

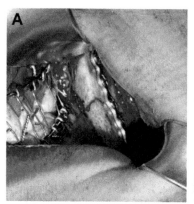
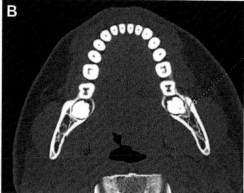

Fig. 4. (*A, B*) Titanium bone plate and screws used for intraoral ORIF of mandibular left angle fracture with cone-beam CT with fracture noted by dotted arrow.

may permit early mobilization of the TMJ and maintain mandibular range of motion. The use of bioresorbable plating technology with polyglycolic or poly-L-lactic plates and screws that resorb by hydrolysis may be used in the pediatric trauma population due to rapid healing potential and need for short-term fixation.[7] (**Fig. 4**)

SOFT TISSUE INJURES

Soft tissue injuries are extremely common in the pediatric population and make up most facial trauma consultations in the emergency setting. These injuries include but are not limited to lacerations, bites, scrapes, thermal and chemical burns. It is important for the evaluating practitioner to recognize the injury modality for proper treatment to be rendered. Most of these injuries are treated in the clinic or emergency department; however, large soft tissue injuries or tissue avulsion are best treated in the operating room. Thorough exploration of the area to check for damage to underlying structures such as the cranial nerve VII (facial) that supplies motor innervation to the muscles of facial expression should be checked by having the patient wrinkle the forehead, close the eyes tightly, or pucker the commissure of the lip on the side of the laceration. Any facial nerve deficits should be documented with possible referral for microsurgical repair by a trained specialist if warranted. In addition, any extensive bleeding vessels should be isolated and cauterized or suture ligated to prevent hematoma formation and possible infection. Delayed or temporary closure of facial lacerations should be considered if there are underlying displaced facial fractures appropriate for ORIF at a later time by access through the preexisting laceration.

Lacerations to facial region should be noted during the examination process previously mentioned. It is important to perform a thorough examination of the scalp and face and clean any dried blood with a wet sponge. It is common to find multiple lacerations, as they can be hidden under dried blood and hair. It is helpful to approach the treatment of facial lacerations in a stepwise fashion. The primary step should be assessing if the pediatric patient will be amenable to repair with local anesthesia or will need sedation. In many instances, sedation may be necessary for adequate repair. Intravenous ketamine is often used as an anesthetic, as there is no cardiac or respiratory depressive activities. Second, the practitioner should administer local anesthetic for analgesia during the repair. Some practitioners will advocate for topical anesthetics such as L.E.T. (lidocaine, epinephrine, tetracaine) and EMLA cream (eutectic mixture of local anesthesia with lidocaine and prilocaine) for repair of small lacerations. Lidocaine with epinephrine is used for local anesthesia in the face and scalp regions without concern for tissue ischemia or necrosis. After local anesthesia is injected, the laceration should be rinsed with copious amounts of saline to remove clots and gross debris and then rinsed with dilute one-tenth mixture of povidone iodine (Betadine) and sterile saline for disinfection of the wound.[8] The wound edges then can be sharply debrided of ragged or devitalized tissue with scissors for an esthetic wound closure. Contaminated or dirty facial lacerations should receive antibiotic coverage usually with penicillin VK for intraoral wounds, or amoxicillin and clavulanate potassium, doxycycline, or cefuroxime for extraoral wounds[8] (**Fig. 5**).

In selection of suture type, there are a few different factors to consider. First would be to assess if the wound will require a multiple-layered closure. Some suture types are better suited for the buried layer and others for skin closure. Another factor would be laceration location, as facial and scalp lacerations can require a different suture type than intraoral lacerations. A third factor would be the use of either resorbable or nonresorbable suture. Resorbable sutures initiate an inflammatory reaction that in turn leads to their degradation. Some suture types, such as chromic gut, cause a significant inflammatory response and thus are not suited for deep layer closure. Suture such as poliglecaprone (Monocryl) and polyglactin (Vicryl) cause minimal inflammatory response and are well-suited for deep layers.[9] For skin closure, 5–0 or 6–0 fast gut or

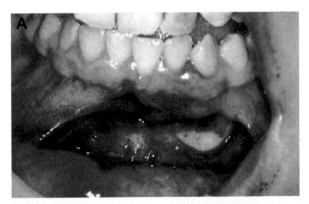

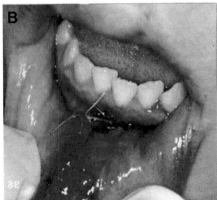
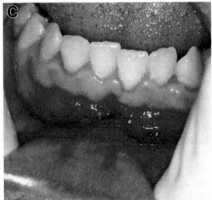

Fig. 5. (*A–C*) Lacerations in the vestibular area, sutured and 2-week follow-up.

polypropylene (Prolene) sutures are good choices.[9] However, it can be advantageous to use resorbable sutures in the pediatric population, as these patients may not cooperate for suture removal. Scalp lacerations are often closed with skin staples, which is quick and easy, although removal in some pediatric patients may require deep sedation or general anesthesia.

Through-and-through lip lacerations are fairly common soft tissue injuries. These lacerations should be closed in a layered manner with attention to initial alignment of the vermillion border of the lip to prevent a noticeable cosmetic defect. A layered closure then is performed from inside out with closure of the oral mucosa, irrigation of the wound to rinse out saliva and bacteria, and then subsequent closure of the orbicularis oris muscle, subcutaneous tissue, and then skin of the lips. Many smaller lacerations that are not full thickness can be treated with skin glue, 2-octyl cyanoacrylate (Dermabond), although its low strength may possibly result in wound dehiscence or breakdown[9] (**Fig. 6**).

Bite wounds from animals or even human bites may be encountered on the face and are treated differently from traumatic lacerations. Antibiotic coverage for most bites uses extended-spectrum amoxicillin-clavulanate (Augmentin) as a primary choice.[10,11] Clindamycin plus levofloxacin or trimethoprim-sulfamethoxazole is an alternative in the patient with a penicillin allergy.[10,11]

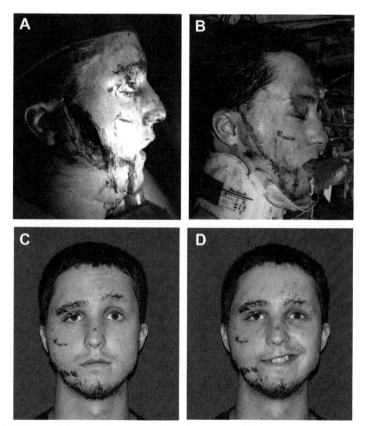

Fig. 6. (*A–D*) Layered closure of adolescent facial lacerations following automobile accident and patient ejected through the windshield. (*D*) with right facial nerve paresis secondary to injury.

Wound debridement and irrigation are important steps in laceration repair, especially in the case of a bite wound. Aggressive debridement of any devitalized tissue is warranted, and copious irrigation with saline to rinse out debris and bacteria is important to lower the chance of infection.

Primary versus delayed closure of bite wounds depends if the bite wounds are narrow and deep. This can make adequate irrigation and debridement of the wound extremely difficult. In these cases, it is best to plan for a delayed closure, as primary closure could trap pathogens deep in the wound and not allow for wound healing.

Rabies/tetanus immunization status should be reviewed for the patient and booster dosing administered if warranted.

DENTAL INJURIES AND DENTOALVEOLAR FRACTURES

Dentoalveolar injuries are common pediatric and adolescent facial injuries and represent 5% of all injuries. Approximately 25% of all school children experience dental trauma, with most injuries occurring before age 19.[12] Luxation injuries are the most common traumatic dental injury in primary teeth, and crown fractures are the most common injuries in permanent teeth.[12] The force directed to a tooth or transmitted through the perioral soft tissue may result in dentoalveolar injuries that may involve the teeth and/or associated alveolar bone.

The following evaluation and treatment protocols are referenced from the latest and comprehensive International Association of Dental Traumatology (IADT) Guidelines 2020 in an open access format.[12] The IADT Guidelines are updated based on current dental literature using EMBASE, MEDLINE, PUBMED, Scopus, and Cochrane Databases for Systematic Reviews from 1996 to 2019 and search of the journal, *Dental Traumatology*, from 2000 to 2019. The goal of these guidelines is to provide information for the immediate or urgent care of traumatic dental injuries with the understanding some follow-up treatment may require secondary or tertiary interventions involving dental and medical specialists experienced in dental trauma. The IADT updated guideline information represents the best evidence-based available literature and expert opinions with the belief that the application of these guidelines can maximize the probability of favorable outcomes.[12]

Dental and dentoalveolar injuries should be evaluated and treated promptly for optimal outcomes, especially related to avulsed teeth. As with other facial injuries, a thorough history should be obtained, including the following: who (age of the patient); what (how the injury occurred); where (clean or contaminated environment); when (time of the injury); overall health of the patient including medications and allergies; any central nervous system (CNS)-related symptoms; any malocclusions; and any record of avulsed or fractured teeth at the trauma site.[13]

Age of the patient is important, as immature permanent teeth with open apices have greater capacity for healing without pulpal degeneration requiring endodontic therapy. Time of the injury related to tooth reimplantation is important. Clean versus dirty environment and need for antibiotics or tetanus prophylaxis should be investigated. How the injury occurred: severity of the trauma, possible other injuries, and possible child abuse considerations should be considered.

What treatment has been provided, if any? Possible tooth replantation and storage of avulsed teeth also are considerations.

Missing or fractured teeth should be accounted for, with possible radiographs of the facial and dentoalveolar areas, possible imaging of the chest or abdomen to rule out swallowed or aspirated missing or fractured teeth (**Fig. 7**).

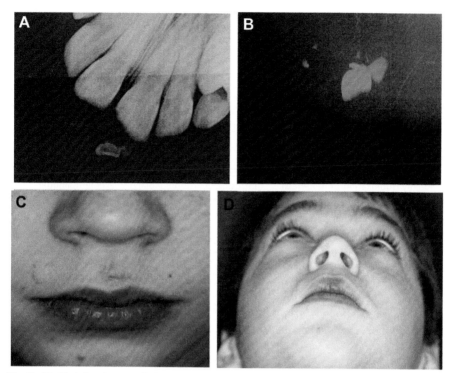

Fig. 7. (*A–D*) Following tooth fracture, fragments were embedded in the patient's lip.

CNS-related symptoms such as nausea, vomiting, headache, confusion, visual changes, amnesia, or loss of consciousness warrant immediate referral and evaluation at a pediatric emergency room. Any malocclusion, possible subluxated tooth, possible dentoalveolar fracture, or jaw fracture require imaging/scans and prompt treatment.

Clinical examination of the facial bones, surrounding soft tissue, oral cavity and structures, and maxilla and mandible, including the alveolar process, should be completed. A thorough dental examination also should be completed regarding tooth or crown fracture, possible pulpal exposure, displacement of teeth, tooth mobility, and percussion sensitivity with periapical or periodontal ligament involvement.

Radiographic examination of involved teeth usually with periapical, panoramic, or possible occlusal films should be completed. Radiographic evaluation of tooth/root fracture, extrusion or intrusion, condition of the periapical bone, root formation, pulp chamber, and any prior endodontic treatment, dentoalveolar fractures, and tooth fragments or foreign debris within the soft tissue should be performed.

Use of the classification of Sanders and colleagues for dentoalveolar injuries is useful to document the extent of injuries and treatment[14] (**Table 2**).

PERMANENT DENTITION DENTAL INJURIES AND DENTOALVEOLAR FRACTURES

Treatment guidelines for dental injuries and dentoalveolar fractures of the permanent dentition are provided again by the IADT guidelines for the management of traumatic dental injuries: 1. Fractures and luxations (**Table 3**).[15]

Table 2
Classification of dentoalveolar injuries

Dentoalveolar Injury	Definition
Crown craze or crack	Crack or incomplete fracture of the enamel without loss of tooth structure
Horizontal or vertical crown fracture	Confined to enamel; enamel and dentin involved; enamel, dentin, and exposed pulp; horizontal or vertical fracture; oblique fracture
Crown-root fracture	No pulp involvement
Horizontal root fracture	Involving apical third; involving middle third; involving cervical third; horizontal or vertical
Mobility (subluxation or looseness)	Intrusion; extrusion; labial displacement; lingual displacement; lateral displacement
Avulsion	Complete displacement of tooth from its socket
Alveolar process fracture	Fracture of alveolar bone in the presence or absence of a tooth or teeth

Data from Sanders B, Brady FA, Johnson R: Injuries.Sanders B. Pediatric Oral and Maxillofacial Surgery.1979.Mosby St Louis, MO.

Treatment of dentoalveolar injuries is based on the clinical examination, radiographs, age and medical condition of the patient, and experience of the dental provider. Some pediatric patients are able to be treated in the office with local anesthesia, whereas younger patients or patients with more complex injuries may require further imaging with cone-beam CT scan or medical CT scan and deep sedation or general anesthesia either in an outpatient facility or hospital setting.

Crown craze lines or cracks limited to enamel with no direct pulpal involvement are usually observed and reevaluated periodically to rule out pulpal or periapical involvement. Crown fractures involving enamel or into dentin may require pulpal protection with calcium hydroxide and restoration.

Tooth with a pulpal exposure that is small may have calcium hydroxide pulp capping and restorative treatment with periodic pulpal evaluation and endodontic treatment initiated if the pulp becomes nonvital. Teeth with large pulpal exposures should generally have endodontic treatment initiated unless the apex is immature, and then pulp

Table 3
Splinting durations for the permanent dentition

Type of Injury	2 Weeks	4 Weeks	4 Months
Subluxation	X (If splinted)		
Extrusion	X		
Lateral luxation		X	
Intrusion		X	
Avulsion	X		
Root fracture (apical 1/3 and middle 1/3)		X	
Root fracture (cervical 1/3)			X
Alveolar fracture		X	

Data from Levin LL, Day PF, Hicks L, et. al. International Association of Dental Traumatology guidelines for the management of traumatic dental injuries: General introduction. Dental Traumatology 2020; 36: 309-313.

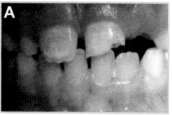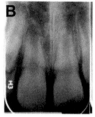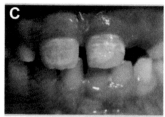

Fig. 8. (*A–C*) Horizontal crown fracture of enamel and dentin; periapical radiograph of the maxillary permanent central incisors with open apices; composite restoration on maxillary left permanent central incisor.

capping with calcium hydroxide and glass ionomer over the exposed dentin, and then a composite restoration completed. Once the apexification is complete following pulp capping, endodontic therapy is then initiated. For a more detailed description of direct pulp capping, see the Adriana Modesto Vieira and Herbert L. Ray's Jr article, "Pediatric Endodontic Treatment of Adolescent Patient," in this issue.

Crown-root fractures treatment depends on the level of the fracture and if there is pulpal involvement and enough tooth structure above the cementoenamel junction (CEJ) to restore the tooth. Teeth with fractures below the CEJ and below the level of the bone are generally nonrestorable and should be extracted with possible immediate implant placement or socket preservation grafting for staged implant placement (**Fig. 8**).

Horizontal root fractures may be treated if the fracture is in the middle to apical third of the root with flexible splinting for approximately 4 weeks for dentinal bridging. Fractures in the cervical third of the tooth close to the gingival margins or CEJ should be extracted.

Teeth with slight mobility may be treated with removal from occlusion and no direct chewing function to allow the reattachment of the tooth and periodic reevaluation of the tooth.

Subluxated teeth with loosening without displacement of the tooth normally require no treatment. If there is excess mobility of the subluxated teeth, stabilize with passive and flexible splinting using stainless steel wire up to 0.4 mm for up to 2 weeks with monitoring of the pulpal vitality.[15]

Displaced teeth that are extruded are treated usually with manual repositioning followed by splinting for 2 weeks and periodic reevaluation for possible endodontic treatment. The clinician must be aware that labial or lingual displacement or lateral displacement may be associated with fracture of adjacent alveolar bone, which may require stabilization with flexible splinting for approximately 4 weeks to promote alveolar bone healing. Intruded teeth should be allowed to re-erupt independent of the degree of intrusion. If the tooth does not erupt within 8 weeks, surgically reposition the tooth and flexible splint for 4 weeks. Intruded teeth with a closed apex generally will require endodontic therapy within 2 weeks.[15]

Avulsed teeth are best managed by the IADT guidelines for the management of traumatic dental injuries: 2. Avulsion of permanent teeth.[13,16]

Avulsed teeth out of the socket have an overall guarded prognosis; replantation at the time of the accident as soon as possible is optimal to prevent desiccation of the periodontal ligament (PDL) cells and pulpal degeneration. Length of time out of the socket is critical, with PDL cells nonviable after 30 minutes. Teeth should be rinsed with milk or saline and replanted as soon as possible by holding the tooth by the crown. Teeth out of the socket for more than 60 minutes have a poor prognosis

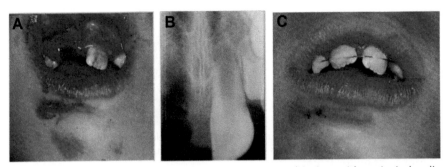

Fig. 9. (A–C) Avulsion of maxillary right permanent central incisor with periapical radiograph illustrating trauma. Light wire passive splint placed to stabilize tooth.

because of PDL necrosis, and resulting ankylosis and root resorption often will occur.[16] There may be some benefit of maintaining esthetics and function and alveolar bone contour by replanting the tooth, as the tooth always can be extracted later with time for planning of tooth replacement options.

Regarding extraoral storage of an avulsed tooth, the best medium is milk (due to protein and electrolytes), Hank's balanced salt solution (Save-A-Tooth Preservation Kit) is second best, then saliva, followed by saline as transport media.[16] Hypotonic tap water should not be used for tooth storage. The tooth socket should be grossly intact and is replanted following rinsing the root and socket gently with saline. The socket should not be curetted to remove the clot and not to damage PDL cells. Teeth should be splinted with a hygienic acid-etch composite and wire splint for 2 weeks to allow reattachment of the tooth/teeth. The less rigid the splint, such as with a passive flexible wire or nylon fishing line, and less splinting time, generally the better the prognosis for the tooth with less ankylosis and external root resorption occurring. Consideration for soaking the tooth with Hank's balanced salt solution for 30 minutes to rehydrate the PDL may be considered. The use of topical antibiotics for 5 minutes to inhibit pulpal bacterial growth and promote revascularization has not been proven beneficial in human studies.[16] Systemic antibiotics with amoxicillin or penicillin, if the patient is not allergic, should be prescribed due to possible contamination of the PDL of the tooth. The tetanus status of the patient should be determined. Root canal therapy should be initiated within 2 weeks after replantation (Fig. 9).

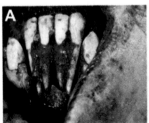
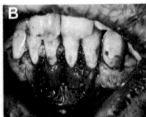
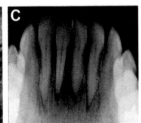

Fig. 10. (A–C) Dentoalveolar fractures.

DENTOALVEOLAR FRACTURES

Fracture of the dental alveolus may occur with dental-related trauma. The alveolar process and teeth may fracture as a unit containing 1 or more teeth. The dentoalveolar segment containing the involved teeth is mobile and moves as a unit with finger pressure. The treatment involves manually repositioning the dentoalveolar segment into the correct anatomic location and splinting the teeth and dentoalveolar segment as a unit commonly with an acid-etched wire or arch bar splint for approximately 4 weeks for osseous healing of the bone.[13] If the dentoalveolar segment is large, referral should be made to an oral and maxillofacial surgeon for intraoral open fracture reduction and possible use of miniplate and screw fixation of the bone segment. Endodontic treatment of the involved teeth should be initiated within 2 weeks of the initial injury to decrease the chance of inflammation resulting in ankylosis or external root resorption (**Fig. 10**).

Regarding the treatment of traumatic dental injuries with splinting, the duration of splinting is variable depending on the dental injury. The IADT provides a nice summary table regarding splinting duration for the permanent dentition.[12]

The treatment of orofacial trauma in the adolescent population is challenging, but also can be a rewarding experience for the trained clinician. Following a systematic approach, the patient is stabilized medically, then progresses to the treatment of any facial fractures. Soft tissue management follows and finally the dental-related injuries are evaluated and treated. Long-term follow-up is necessary to monitor healing, any subsequent injuries, and failures of treatment.

CLINICS CARE POINTS

- Adolescent facial and dental-related trauma occurs frequently in the pediatric population, especially during the adolescent period.
- Initial evaluation of the medical condition must be completed and treated as a priority.
- Facial fractures may be monitored and managed by conservation means or closed reduction techniques.
- Soft tissue injuries should be repaired with debridement and irrigation of the wounds.
- Once the patient is medically stable, then dental-related trauma should be evaluated and treated.

DISCLOSURE

The authors have nothing to disclose.

REFERENCES

1. Braun TL, Xue AS, Maricevich RS. Differences in the management of pediatric facial trauma. Semin Plast Surg 2017;31:118–22.
2. Chang MC, Stewart RM, Rotondo MF, et al. National trauma data bank pediatric report 2016. Chicago, (IL): American College of Surgeons; 2016. p. 1–128.
3. Lee LK, Fleisher GR. Trauma management: approach to the unstable child. UpToDate 2020;1–61.
4. RadilogyInfo.Org. Radiation Dose in Xrays and CT scans. Oakbrook, (IL): Radiological Society of North America, Proceedings; 2019.
5. Radiation Risks and pediatric computed tomography (CT): a guide for health care providers. Bethesda, (MD): National Cancer Institute position paper 2021; 1-6.

6. Hatef DA, Cole PD, Hollier LH Jr. Contemporary management of pediatric facial fractures. Curr Opinions Otolaryngol Head Neck Surg 2009;17:308–14.

7. Eppley BL, Morales L, Wood R, et al. Resorbable PLLA-PGA plate and screw fixation in pediatric craniofacial surgery: clinical experience in 1883 patients. Plast Reconstr Surg 2004;114(4):850–6.

8. Parish KD, Cothran VE, Young CC. Facial soft tissue injuries medication: antibiotics0. Medscape 2021;1–4.

9. Dunn DL. Ethicon wound closure manual. Raritan, (NJ): Ethicon Inc.; 2005.

10. Baddour LM, Harper M, Wolfson AB. Animal bites (dogs, cats, and other animals): evaluation and management. UpToDate 2021;1–17.

11. Baddor LM, Harper M, Wolfson AB. Human bites: evaluation and management. UpToDate 2021;1–13.

12. Levin LL, Day PF, Hicks L, et al. International Association of Dental Traumatology guidelines for the management of traumatic dental injuries: general introduction. Dental Traumatol 2020;36:309–13.

13. Hupp JR, Ellis E, Tucker MR. Contemporary oral and maxillofacial surgery. 7th edition. Philadelphia (PA): Elsevier Inc; 2019.

14. Sanders B, Brady FA, Johnson R, et al. Pediatric oral and maxillofacial surgery. St Louis (MO): Mosby; 1979.

15. Bourguinon C, Cohenca N, Laridsen E, et al. International Association of Dental Traumatology guidelines for the management of traumatic dental injuries: 1. Fractures and luxations. Dental Traumatol 2020;36:314–30.

16. Foud AF, Abbot PV, Tsilingardis G, et al. International Association of Dental Traumatology guidelines for the management of traumatic dental injuries: 2. Avulsion of permanent teeth. Dental Truamatology 2020;36:331–42.

Evaluation and Management of Impacted Teeth in the Adolescent Patient

Bryce Hartman, DDS[a], Edward C. Adlesic, MS, DMD[b],*

KEYWORDS

- Introduction and incidence • Classification of impacted teeth
- Indications and contraindications • Technique

KEY POINTS

- Third molars are the most frequently encountered impacted teeth followed by maxillary canines and mandibular premolars
- CBCT imaging is commonly used to identify location and proximity to surrounding teeth, inferior alveolar nerve, and the maxillary sinus.
- Retention of impacted teeth increase long-term morbidities: periodontal disease, pericoronitis, odontogenic cysts and tumors, root resorption of adjacent teeth, and unexplained pain.
- Postoperative morbidity is more frequent in patients beyond age 25 years.

INTRODUCTION/INCIDENCE/CAUSE

Identification and proper management of impacted teeth should be a useful tool in the dentist's armamentarium. Using evidence-based data to support recommended treatments and knowing proper classification systems can assist the dentist coordinate proper patient care. This article provides the pediatric dentist useful information to know when to obtain imaging, when to refer to an oral surgeon, and when to avoid treatment. Indications for impacted teeth treatment, contraindications, expected postoperative course, and potential complications are also reviewed.

A tooth is considered impacted when it fails to erupt within the expected time period and can no longer be reasonably expected to do so. Third molars are most commonly impacted and are extensively discussed; however, maxillary canines and mandibular premolars are the next most frequent impacted teeth. Of particular importance to

[a] Oral and Maxillofacial Surgery, University of Pittsburgh Medical Center, 180 Couch Rd., Suite 250, Pittsburgh, PA 15241, USA; [b] Department of Oral and Maxillofacial Surgery, Department of Dental Anesthesiology, University of Pittsburgh School of Dental Medicine, G32 Salk Hall, 3501 Terrace Street, Pittsburgh, PA 15261, USA
* Corresponding author.
E-mail address: eca17@pitt.edu

Dent Clin N Am 65 (2021) 805–814
https://doi.org/10.1016/j.cden.2021.07.003
0011-8532/21/© 2021 Elsevier Inc. All rights reserved.

dental.theclinics.com

pediatric dentists, true impaction of primary teeth is uncommon. Unerupted primary teeth likely are secondary to absent successor permanent teeth typically due to syndromes, rather than local processes, such as inadequate arch length.[1] There are many syndromes associated with multiple impacted teeth, including but not limited to cleidocranial dysplasia, Down syndrome, and Gardner syndrome.[2] The most common impacted supernumerary tooth is the mesiodens, followed by the supernumerary maxillary incisor, fourth molar, and mandibular premolar.[3] Multiple impacted primary teeth should therefore alert the pediatric dentist to systemic consideration.

This article focuses on classification schemes to aid in communication, the role of imaging in treatment options, the timing of treatment, and indications and contraindications for extractions. With increased understanding, pediatric dentists can better anticipate difficult cases and ensure that patients are being treated within the proper time frame, using scrutinized literature to support these decisions rather than arbitrary personal experience. We also focus on pearls and pitfalls of the technique of third molar extractions, potential complications, and expected postoperative course.

CLASSIFICATIONS

When describing impacted third molars, classification schemes can aid the pediatric dentist in communication. A commonly referred scheme is the Pell and Gregory classification, which is used to describe the position of impacted lower third molars. As depicted in **Fig. 1**, classes A, B, and C relate the height of the impacted third molar's occlusal plane to the mandibular second molar. In class A the impacted third molar's occlusal plane is even with the second molar's occlusal plane. In class B the impacted third molar's occlusal plane is below the second molar's occlusal plane but above the cement-enamel junction (CEJ) of the second molar. In class C the impacted third molar's occlusal plane is below the CEJ of the second molar. Classes 1, 2, and 3 indicate the anterior-posterior relationship of the impacted third molar to the anterior ramus. Class 1 indicates there is sufficient space between the ascending ramus and second molar for eventual eruption. A class 2 impacted third molar's distal crown is

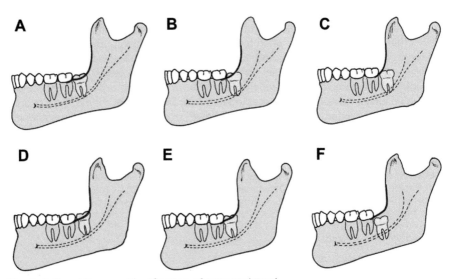

Fig. 1. Pell and Gregory Classification of Impacted Teeth.

covered by bone of the ascending ramus, whereas a class 3 impacted third molar's entire crown is totally embedded within the ramus. As the classification advances from 1 to 3 and from A to C, the extraction can be anticipated to be more difficult.

A more commonly used classification system, and potentially more practical, classifies the third molars based on the nature of the overlying tissue and directionality; this can be used to refer to maxillary and mandibular third molars. Soft tissue impacted teeth have a height of contour that is occlusal to the surrounding alveolus, but still remain covered by soft tissue. Partial bony impacted teeth have eruption impeded by soft tissue but have a height of contour below the surrounding alveolus. Similarly, complete bony impacted teeth are those that are completely embedded within bone. Last, Winter classification is used to describe the directionality of impacted third molars in relation to the vertical axis of the adjacent second molars: mesial angular, distal angular, horizontal, vertical, etc.

IMAGING

Clinical examination and adjunct imaging can provide diagnosis of an impacted tooth. Routinely, a panorex is initially provided to evaluate the position and stage of development of the impacted teeth. Sometimes, an in-office dental cone beam computed tomography (CBCT) is completed to provide a 3-dimensional analysis of impacted tooth position as it relates to vital structures. In the case of impacted mandibular third molars, the CBCT will allow for evaluation of these teeth in relation to the inferior alveolar nerve, as well as thickness of adjacent lingual cortex. Panorex findings suggesting close approximation of mandibular third molars include darkening, narrowing, and deflection of the third molar root and diversion of the inferior alveolar canal.[4] Of these findings, however, darkening of the third molar root caries the highest relative risk of inferior alveolar nerve damage. The information provided by a CBCT can often dictate treatment, including extraction versus coronectomy. Studies have shown that a preoperative CBCT influenced the treatment plan for 12% of cases.[5] Other findings in CBCTs can change treatment plans other than coronectomy versus extraction of mandibular third molars. Severe external resorption observed in CBCTs was the main decisive factor for removing the second instead of third molar when considering maxillary third molar preoperative evaluation.[6]

CBCT imaging also has a role in evaluating other impacted teeth, to aid in surgical access. Knowing whether an impacted maxillary canine is buccal or lingual to root apices of adjacent erupted teeth allows the surgeon to determine whether to access the impacted tooth from the palate or buccal vestibule. Also, the CBCT can determine feasibility of eruption once impacted canine is exposed. Studies have shown a correlation of panorex findings and CBCT-confirmed labial or palatal tooth positioned. For instance, if the panorex shows a horizontally positioned maxillary canine, the CBCT will indicate that the tooth is on the palate. It is suggested to obtain a CBCT to confirm.[7]

TIMING OF TREATMENT

Appropriate treatment of impacted teeth can be guided by dentists, with particular emphasis placed on timing of treatment. Ideal timing allows for easier surgery, which in turn allows for improved patient outcomes and recovery. In 2007, the American Association of Oral and Maxillofacial Surgeons created a task force to review literature with regard to impacted third molar removal, releasing the "White Paper on Third Molar Data." The data released in this paper guides official treatment recommendations and provides proper indications for third molar removal. Of particular importance to pediatric dentists are conclusions from "The Effects of Age on Various Parameters Relating to Third Molars." Multiple studies found that postoperative morbidity following third molar removal is higher in patients older than 25 years (pain, swelling, food impaction, purulent discharge). Postoperative periodontal defects, namely increased pocket depths, occur twice as often (51%) in patients older than age 26 compared to patients younger than 25. Caries in erupted third molars increases in prevalence with increasing age. After age 25, it is apparent that all potential surgical risks associated with third molar surgery have an increased incidence. A study of 4004 patients showed a 1.5 times likelihood of a complication if the patient had third molars removed at age greater than 25 years with generalized increasing risks with age through 65 years. The document identified a germectomy as the removal of an impacted tooth that has one-third or less of root formation and a discernible periodontal ligament. Although dental development varies patient to patient, studies with patients aged 9 to 17 years reported significant decreases in alveolar osteitis, nerve involvement, second molar damage, and infection.[8]

NON–THIRD MOLAR IMPACTED TEETH

Pediatric dentist providers also must be prepared for the management and timing considerations for non–third molar impactions. Surgical uprighting of a mesioangular impacted mandibular second molar is often required to aid in eruption. This procedure will usually require removal of the adjacent impacted third molar. It is not necessary to remove buccal bone or place a bracket. The procedure is best performed after two-thirds of root development is completed. At this stage, the risk of root fracture is minimal. Although the procedure has been performed when root development is complete, the incidence of subsequent pulpal necrosis or calcification is increased.[9,10]

Another non–third molar impacted tooth consideration is the surgical exposure and often bonding of impacted maxillary canines. Given the eruption sequence, these teeth often require additional procedures to facilitate eruption. For non–third molar impacts, the most desirable treatment outcome is eruption of the tooth into its normal, functional position in the dental arch. The most common example of this is the impacted maxillary canine. Eruption is often facilitated by a combined surgical and orthodontic approach, exposure and bond. This procedure includes surgical access to the impacted canine, including bone removal, but not to the level of the CEJ. Once accessed, an orthodontic bracket and chain are bonded to the impacted tooth. Orthodontic forces are then applied to facilitate eruption. Exposure should be carried out conservatively so that only enough bone and soft tissue are removed to place an orthodontic bracket. Damaging effects to the periodontium have been shown to be more frequent with exposure of the CEJ.[1]

INDICATIONS

Impacted teeth that are not able to function represent potential adverse outcomes. Given the above-mentioned White Paper conclusions, impacted third molars should be removed prophylactically to avoid pathologic problems that result from impacted teeth, including periodontitis, pericoronitis, odontogenic cysts and tumors, root resorption of adjacent teeth, jaw fracture, and unexplained pain. One critical indication for extraction is to prevent pathologic condition. Curran and colleagues[11] studied 2646 lesions involving impacted third molars and concluded that 33% of those lesions showed significant pathology. The most common pathologic condition was dentigerous cyst (28.4%), followed by odontogenic keratocyst (3%), odontoma (0.7%), and ameloblastoma (0.5%).[11]

CONTRAINDICATIONS

One of the most controversial issues regarding impacted mandibular third molars is their role in postorthodontic therapy anterior crowding. Although this is a common thought process among practitioners, the data do not support this claim. Anterior incisor crowding is associated with deficient arch length, not the presence of impacted teeth.[10] However, it can be assumed that patients who recently finished orthodontic therapy can still stand to benefit from third molar removal given the anticipated age of such patient and prevention of the aforementioned potential adverse outcomes of impacted teeth. Prophylactic extractions of asymptomatic impacted third molars in individuals older than 35 years, in particular those with other associated risk factors (close approximation to the inferior alveolar nerve, anticipated difficult extractions given Pell and Gregory classification), are contraindicated.

ARMAMENTARIUM

The appropriate armamentarium is a necessity if the practitioner plans to surgically treat impacted teeth. **Fig. 2** shows the basic tray setup for surgical extraction of impacted teeth. Appropriate application of each of these standard instruments is beyond the scope of this article; however, specialized instruments in **Fig. 3** can be further discussed. From left to right, the instruments are a spade elevator, a 46R elevator, a crane elevator, and a 69W chisel. The spade elevator is of particular use in areas with tight interproximal purchase points. While maintaining palatal pressure, the spade can be wedged mesial to maxillary third molars to aid in elevation. The advantage of a 46R elevator is the offset shank that allows the provider to achieve an appropriate angle to elevation. A crane elevator is of particular use when a purchase point is created in a tooth; it can also be applied to the pulp chamber following sectioning mandibular third molars to facilitate delivery. Last, the 69W chisel can function to remove buccal bone overlying a maxillary third molar if the aforementioned bone is too dense for a periosteal to remove enough bone for evaluation and purchase of impacted maxillary third molars.

TECHNIQUE

Once the patient accepts the treatment plan, they are ready for surgery. After adequate local anesthesia is administered, the provider must expose the impacted tooth properly with an understanding of surrounding anatomy; this begins with incision

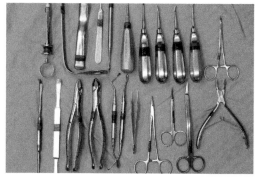

Fig. 2. Oral Surgery Tray Setup.

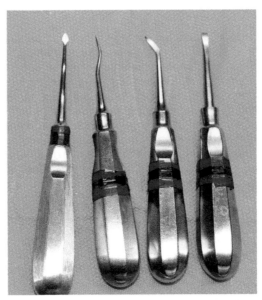

Fig. 3. Elevators (Left to right) Spade, 46R, Crane Pick, Hand Chisel 69W.

design. The most common flap for removal of impacted third molars is an envelope flap, incorporating the sulcus of the erupted first and second molars, and a distal oblique posterior incision. Care must be taken to keep this distal oblique incision over bone; this avoids the potential complication of lingual nerve injury. Otherwise, if the distal incision is carried straight posterior, there is a chance it extends into the sublingual space and damages the lingual nerve. On average the lingual nerve is located approximately 2 mm medial and 2 mm inferior to the height of the lingual cortex. In 10% to 15% of patients, the lingual nerve is immediately adjacent to the height of the lingual cortex. After incision, care must be taken to ensure a subperiosteal dissection is maintained laterally. Increased postoperative swelling and discomfort can be attributed to supraperiosteal dissection.

Once a soft tissue flap has been elevated, and adequate visualization of the surgical field is ensured, the provider must then remove overlying bone. Bone on the occlusal, buccal, and distal surfaces should be removed to properly identify the buccal groove for eventual sectioning. The angulation of the impacted tooth, root morphology, and anticipated degree of difficulty should guide in the initial bone removal; however, generally enough bone should be removed to visualize the CEJ on the buccal and distal surfaces (**Fig. 4**).

For maxillary third molars, bone removal is often unnecessary given the thin nature of the adjacent buccal plate. However, when necessary, adequate exposure can be accomplished with the use of a periosteal elevator to flake off the thinner buccal plate. An alternative technique uses a 69W hand chisel elevator to remove bone over the tooth.

Once properly exposed, the next step is to section the tooth to provide a path of draw for elevation and extraction. There are a couple of guiding principles to aid in a successful split—sectioning the tooth into equal mesial and distal segments. First, the buccal groove must be properly identified to guide the mesial/distal extension of the sectioning. Second, the provider must keep the drill oriented along the long axis

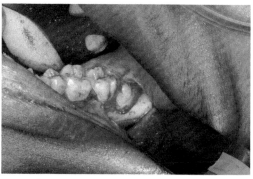

Fig. 4. Surgical Exposure of Impacted Third Molar.

of the tooth, although horizontally impacted teeth are often an exception to this principle. Last, the tooth is only sectioned three-fourths of the way through toward the lingual aspect; this allows for the lingual plate to be preserved without damage and therefore avoid lingual nerve injury (**Fig. 5**).

The use of a wide, straight elevator can finish propagation of the split. The distal half of the tooth should be delivered first; therefore, sufficient distal bone adjacent to the impacted tooth must be removed. Attempting to deliver the mesial half first should be avoided because there is insufficient space given the proximity to the second molar and the remaining distal half. Often, the crown of the distal half is sectioned at the CEJ, as was the case in **Fig. 6**. Removing just the distal crown allows for space to deliver the mesial half of the tooth, before returning to the distal root to complete the extraction. A double-ended curette can then be used to exfoliate any residual follicle, which is typically the case for complete bony impacted third molars. Often a bone file is used to smooth any irregularities from surgical bone removal. Last, the site is irrigated with particular attention to the subperiosteal flap laterally before soft tissue reapproximation, typically with resorbable chromic gut suture.

COMPLICATIONS

Recovery following impacted tooth removal can vary from patient to patient, depending on the complexity of extraction. However, an average postoperative timeline can

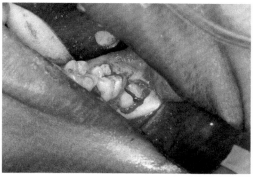

Fig. 5. Crown Sectioned.

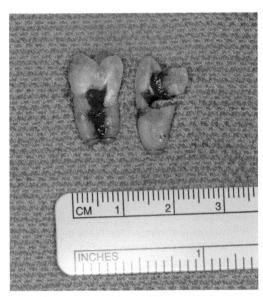

Fig. 6. Tooth was sectioned into 3 pieces for excision.

help identify potential complications. For example, discomfort in postoperative day 1 or 2 is expected. Discomfort occurring within postoperative days 4 to 7 could indicate alveolar osteitis, also known as dry socket. In a prospective study involving 3760 patients older than 25 years the incidence of localized alveolar osteitis was 12% in mandibular molars. Other complication rates were infection, 1%; inferior alveolar nerve injury, 1.1%–1.7%; and lingual nerve injury, 0.3%.[12] Postoperative antibiotics are recommended for patients undergoing contaminated, long-duration surgery, because studies have shown a decrease in alveolar osteitis with a 3-day course of antibiotics.[13] Nerve injury identification is also a time-sensitive finding. Axonotmesis, or traction injury, is injury to the axons and their myelin sheath, but the endoneurium, perineurium, and epineurium remain intact. This injury is the most common type of nerve injury during dentoalveolar surgery, and complete recovery occurs typically within 12 weeks.

CORONAVIRUS DISEASE 2019 IMPACT

In light of the ongoing global pandemic, there have been changes to treatment of impacted teeth. Given that many impacted teeth require bone removal via a surgical hand piece, there is a higher risk of transmission of respiratory aerosols. Proper personal protective equipment (PPE) is recommended, including the routine use of N95 respirators. For those practitioners who are unable to pass an N95 fit test, a powered air-purifying respirator is then recommended. Up-to-date, efficient ventilation systems and negative pressure rooms help to decrease potential spread via aerosols. Practitioners should follow official state and American Dental Association guidelines to help guide PPE and office protocols. Although the treatment of impacted teeth is often considered elective, there should not be a delay in treatment given the time-sensitive nature of these procedures. As outlined previously, increasing age is associated with an increased risk of complications.

SUMMARY

Proper management of impacted teeth is a useful tool for the dentist. Proper classification and terminology can aid in communication and allow the practitioner to anticipate more difficult cases. The indications and benefits of extracting impacted teeth prophylactically outweigh the potential complications. The research and data culminated from the "White Paper on Third Molar Data" resonate this claim. Proper instrument armamentarium and surgical technique ensure success for the practitioner and aid in improved patient outcomes.

CLINICS CARE POINTS

- Third molars are the most common impacted tooth.
- Panorex imaging is the standard radiograph used in the evaluation of impacted teeth. When nerve position is questionable, a Cone Beam Computed Tomograph is indicated.
- Surgical complications are more common after age 26.

DISCLOSURE

The authors have nothing to disclose.

REFERENCES

1. Bianchi SD, Roccuzzo M. Primary impaction of primary teeth: a review and report of three cases. J Clin Pediatr Dent 1991;15:165–8.
2. Zeitler D. Management of impacted teeth other than third molars. Oral Maxillofac Surg Clin North Am 1993;5(1):95–103.
3. Kaban LB, Troulis MJ. Dentoalveolar surgery. In: Kaban T, editor. Pediatric oral and maxillofacial surgery. Philadelphia: WB Saunders; 2004. p. 125–45.
4. Sedaghatfar M, August MA, Dodson TB. Panoramic radiographic findings as predictors of inferior alveolar nerve exposure following third molar extraction. J Oral Maxillofac Surg 2005;63:3–7.
5. Matzen H, Schou S, Wenzel A. Influence of cone beam CT on treatment plan before surgical intervention of mandibular third molars and impact of radiographic factors on deciding on coronectomy verses surgical removal. Dentomaxillofac Radiol 2013;42(1):98870341.
6. Hermann L, Wenzel A, Schropp L, et al. Impact of CBCT on treatment decision related to surgical removal of impacted maxillary third moars: does CBCT change the surgical approach? Dentomaxillofacial Radiol 2019;48(8): 20190209.
7. Ngo CTT, Fishman LS, Rossouw PE, et al. Correlation between panoramic radiography and cone-beam computed tomography in assessing maxillary impacted canines. Angle Orthod 2018;88(4):384–9.
8. American Association of Oral and Maxillofacial Surgeons. White paper on third molar data. AAOMS Surg Update 2007;21(1):1–20.
9. Dessner S. Surgical uprighting of second molars: rationale and technique. Oral Maxillofac Surg Clin North Am 2002;14(2):201–12.
10. Costello BJ, Mallik AKB, Powers M, et al. Complicated exodontia. In: Fonseca RJ, editor. Oral and maxillofacial sugery, vol. 1. St. Louis: WB Saunders; 2000. p. 240.

11. Curran AE, Damm DD, Drummond JF. Pathologically significant pericoronal lesions in adults: histopathologic evaluation. J Oral Maxillofac Surg 2002;60(6):613–7.
12. Ness GM. Impacted Teeth. In: Waite P, editor. Peterson's principles of oral and maxillofacial surgery. People's Medical Pub. House-USA; 2012. p. 97–123. Chapter 5.
13. Haug RH, Perrott DH, Gonzalez ML, et al. The American Association of oral and maxillofacial surgeons age-related third molar study. J Oral Maxillofac Surg 2005;63(8):1106–14.

Legal and Ethical Issues in Treating Adolescent Patients

Pamela Zarkowski, JD, MPH[a],*, Mert N. Aksu, DDS, JD, MHSA, Cert DPH[b]

KEYWORDS

• Legal • Ethical adolescent dental care • Pediatric legal considerations

KEY POINTS

- The ethical principles of justice, veracity, nonmaleficence, beneficence, and autonomy are essential considerations in interactions with adolescents, parents, and guardians.
- Adolescents are minors; however, state laws vary in the rights given to adolescents, and providers should be familiar with them to protect themselves and their patients.
- Each state has unique laws governing the practice of dentistry and delegation of duties; in addition, it is important to understand professional responsibilities under contract and tort law.
- Decision making should involve the adolescent patient whenever possible and practitioners should understand the complexities of the parent/guardian relationship when making decisions about care.
- Providers must be sensitive to current trends and issues associated with caring for adolescents, risky behaviors, mandated reporting obligations, responsible pain management practices, and mental health wellness.

INTRODUCTION

Respectful, quality oral health care is the goal of all dental care providers (**Boxes 1–3, Table 1**). Care must be guided by legal and ethical principles while considering the unique status of each patient that has matured from a child and has not yet reached adulthood. Knowledge of key concepts and principles guide providers in their interactions, communication, record keeping, and decision making.

The American Academy of Pediatric Dentists provides a framework in its Policy on a Patient's Bill of Rights and Responsibilities, revised in 2019.[1] Patient rights noted include recommendations for:

- Respectful care

[a] University of Detroit Mercy, Office of Academic Administration, 4001 West McNichols, Detroit, MI 48221, USA; [b] University of Detroit Mercy, School of Dentistry, 2700 Martin Luther King Jr. Boulevard, Detroit, MI 48208-2576, USA
* Corresponding author.
E-mail address: zarkowp1@udmercy.edu

Dent Clin N Am 65 (2021) 815–826
https://doi.org/10.1016/j.cden.2021.06.011
0011-8532/21/© 2021 Elsevier Inc. All rights reserved.

dental.theclinics.com

Box 1
Professionalism traits

- Respect for others
- Competence
- Responsibility
- Competence, caring, and compassion
- Maturity and self-awards
- Reliability and responsibility

- Knowledge of the identity of all providers
- Full participation in all decisions related to care
- Accurate, relevant, and easily understood information concerning diagnosis, treatment, and prognosis
- Information about specific procedures and/or treatments, including risks, benefits, and alternatives
- Participating in decision making, including informed refusal
- Privacy
- Confidentiality
- Availability of records

The policy is directed to parents or guardians and patients. The policy outlines patient responsibilities, including an obligation to provide accurate information, transparent communication, and considerate behavior to providers.

The information provided in this article must be considered in light of professional codes of ethics and the laws of each state, including dental practice acts. Knowledge about ethical principles provides a foundation for a more specific discussion about adolescent care and frequently encountered situations.

Furthermore, patient expectations and consumerism in health care have shaped the understanding that dental care will be of high-quality with predictable outcomes and provide patient satisfaction. In addition, the expectation is that patients will have a

---

Box 2
Elements of informed refusal documentation

- The recommended treatment or procedure and justification
- The educational documents, brochures, handouts, or presentations given to or viewed by the patient
- Oral and health risks
- The questions asked and the answers that were provided (by both parties)
- That the patient was informed of the risks of not following the recommendations
- The patient's reasons for refusal
- That the consequences of the refusal were reexplained, and whether the patient still refused the recommended treatment or procedures (note that the patient understood the risks of refusing care)
- Individuals present and signatures of the patient, witness, and provider

---

Box 3
Types of guardianship situations

- Joint guardianship: caregiver shared custody with a parent
- Short-term guardianship or custody: parent appoints person to have temporary control over child
- Standby guardianship: preappointed future guardian steps in after a triggering event
- Limited: powers of guardian limited to those set forth by order
- De facto custody: child's primary caregiver for some time in the parent's absence

---

significant role in directing the decision-making processes. The role of adolescent patients in this process must be navigated depending on the emotional and maturational level of each patient.

ADOLESCENT PATIENTS

The American Academy of Pediatrics divides adolescence into 3 age groups: early (ages 11–14 years), middle (ages 15–17 years), and late (ages 18–21 years).[2] Treating adolescent patients is associated with several considerations. Although, developmentally, adolescence is viewed as the physical, psychosocial, sexual, and intellectual period of transition from childhood to adulthood, there are also transitional legal rights recognized during this time. For instance, routine medical history questions may trigger a right to privacy for minor adolescent patients; in addition, the patient may be able to develop a right to refuse treatment even if the parent insists that the adolescent child receive care. Despite their physical maturity, adolescents may have difficulty communicating and trouble expressing their feelings about dental care and

Table 1
Brief summary of intentional torts with examples

Specific Tort	Description	Example
Assault	The threat of bodily harm to another; there does not have to be physical contact	Waving a syringe in a threatening manner
Battery	Bodily harm without permission	Performing a procedure without the consent of the patient
False imprisonment	Violation of personal liberty through unlawful restraint	Refusing to allow a patient to leave the operator/office
Mental distress	Purposeful cause of anguish	Causing distress to someone in front of another
Defamation of character	Damage caused to a person's reputation either in writing (libel) or spoken (slander)	Making an untrue negative statement about a dental peer
Misrepresentation	Incorrect or false representation	Promising a cure for a dental condition

their willingness to accept the treatment. It may be cognitively and emotionally difficult for an adolescent child to express fear or to understand the long-term consequences of disease processes.

The patients should be involved in the decision process regardless of their status as minors. The American Dental Association (ADA) Principles of Ethics and Code of Professional Conduct (ADA Code) recommends that patients be provided information "in a manner that allows the patient to become involved in treatment decisions."[3] Furthermore, from an ethical perspective, "the dentist's primary obligations include involving patients in treatment decisions in a meaningful way, with due consideration being given to the patient's needs, desires and abilities, and safeguarding the patient's privacy."[3] The degree to which each adolescent patient is engaged and involved requires careful consideration of the individual circumstances, the relationship between the patient and the parent/guardian, complexities of the case, and the patient's previous experience with dental procedures.

Adolescents may present with emerging signs of mental illness and depression. Adolescent patients also may engage in risky behaviors, including tobacco, nicotine, alcohol, and recreational drug use. Sexual activity may result in oral manifestations of sexually transmitted diseases. The legal and ethical considerations associated with the confidentiality of these issues need careful attention. The dental office staff should be sensitive to the confidentiality of patient disclosures during care.

OVERVIEW OF LEGAL AND ETHICAL PRINCIPLES
Ethical Principles

Ethical principles provide a framework for judgment and decision making. The American Dental Association's Principles of Ethics and Code of Conduct, and other professional codes, outline 5 principles and offer commentary (https://www.ada.org/en/about-the-ada/principles-of-ethics-code-of-professional-conduct).

A foundational principle in ethics is nonmaleficence. This principle is commonly known as "Do no harm" and means that the provider's first obligation is to the patient. It is associated with preventing and removing harm. A dental office shows this principle in all activities, ranging from disinfection and sterilization of operatories and equipment, to treatment and patient education.

Beneficence is an obligation to promote each patient's welfare and best interests. Beneficence requires providers to deliver services to their patients and the public at large. A patient's needs, desires, and values are taken into consideration in the dental office setting.

Autonomy is based on respect for an individual. The principle allows individuals to be self-governing and self-directing in their decision making. Providing accurate information related to treatment and treatment outcomes shows a respect for the patient's autonomy in determining whether to accept or decline a treatment plan.

Justice is fairness, an obligation to treat people equitably. This principle applies to patients, colleagues, and society. Dental services should be provided without prejudice.

Veracity is truthfulness and requires a duty to communicate honestly and clearly. It supports a relationship of trust between the provider and the patient critical to the relationship.

Additional ethical principles include confidentiality and fidelity. Confidentiality is an obligation that limits access to information that is provided by a patient to a provider. Fidelity recognizes the special relationship that develops between patients and providers. It may be viewed as providing quality competent care to patients as part of the providers' professional responsibility.

Dental providers are credentialed and licensed to provide care to patients. In addition to adhering to the ethical principles, Integral to their professional standing within their community and among their peers is an expectation that interactions with patients, parents and guardians, and peers will model the following characteristics:

Legal Principles

An understanding of legal principles guides providers in their day-to-day interactions with patients. Dentists can be sued for both criminal and civil violations. Dentists are often concerned about allegations of negligence. Dentists can be guilty of criminal offenses related to sexual misconduct, drug diversion, and fraud. State dental practice acts and legislation may hold dental providers accountable for other actions, including reporting child abuse and child neglect and human trafficking.

Civil Law

There are 2 types of civil law. Tort law is interfering with an individuals' ability to enjoy their persons, privacy, or property. There are 3 types of tort classifications:

- Intentional torts occur when an individual intentionally commits a wrongful act causing harm to another individual. There is a requirement to show that the person committing the tort did so on purpose.
- Unintentional torts occur when there is unintentional harm to a person and a failure to exercise a reasonable standard of care, such as in dental negligence. Four elements are necessary to prove an unintentional tort:
  - A duty is owed to the patient
  - A breach of the duty occurs
  - Patient suffers damages
  - The resulting harm is caused by the breach (causation)

From a legal perspective, third-party payers have a significant role in dental care quality assurance. From the perspective of proper use, ensuring quality outcomes, and documentation of medical necessity, third-party payers are increasingly involved in the review of care. With 37,581,693 minors enrolled in the Children's Health Insurance Program or children enrolled in the Medicaid program in the 50 states,[4] the single most prominent influencer of allegations of improper care stems from utilization reviews.

Third-party payers are incentivized and contractually required to implement quality improvement and utilization review programs. As a result, audits of dental records can result in allegations of improper treatment and overtreatment. These audits are defensible with proper documentation and justification of medical necessity. Absent appropriate documentation, the provider is subject to demands for repayment for unnecessary care, allegations of malpractice, and potential state board action. Third-party payers can extrapolate the value of losses based on a sampling of a subset of patient records. Based on the extrapolation, providers may find themselves responsible for hundreds of thousands of dollars of repayment.

In general, the period for the statute of limitations for malpractice on a minor allows for a claim to be filed for up to 3 years from the date of the alleged injury, or, if the alleged injury is concealed, 3 years from the discovery of the injury, or 6 months from the child's 18th birthday, whichever is longer. There are minor variations in the statute of limitations laws between the various states.

Regarding malpractice claims, the highest risk for settlement relates to anesthesia overdosing, nerve trauma during surgical procedures, malocclusion and subsequent temporomandibular joint dysfunction, and lacerations to the soft tissue. Emerging areas for liability include the need for practitioners to carefully understand and assess the airway and the possible impact of malocclusion on adult obstructive airway apnea, because, left untreated, some malocclusions could create comorbidities with sleep apnea in adults.

Contract law is the second area of civil law. A contract is an agreement between 2 or more consenting and competent parties to do or not to do something for which there is an exchange value, such as payment for services. Dentists have contractual relationships with their patients based on either a written agreement, such as a treatment plan, or the patient's actions of seeking care and the dentist providing the care. The contractual relationship holds the dentist and patient to specific obligations, including delivering competent and timely care by licensed professionals, using acceptable dental materials and techniques, and remaining current and up to date. Because government-sponsored insurance plans cover so many children, it is critical to note that the most important and most significant contract related to the provision of care is the provider agreement that dentists enter into as a part of their insurance participation. These participation agreements set parameters for expectations related to the predictability of the outcomes of care and the need to justify the performance of only medically necessary care. These contracts also prescribe the payment schedule for each procedure and the reasons for payment ineligibility.

Informed Consent and Informed Refusal

To successfully meet the standard of care, a dental provider must fulfill the duties associated with the action performed. A duty is a legal obligation. Duty requires that a provider use care toward others that would protect anyone from unnecessary harm. Dentists, by the nature of their education and licensure, have a variety of duties. Patient care includes assessment, treatment planning, treatment, evaluation of outcomes, and maintenance of oral health.

Informed consent is the patient's right to understand the recommended procedures, risks, and alternatives. The ADA Principles of Ethics and Code of Professional Conduct[3] section 1.A, entitled Patient Involvement, clearly states that the dentist should inform the patient of the proposed treatment and any reasonable alternatives that allow the patient to become involved in treatment decisions. It is the duty of the dentist to obtain consent. Informed consent, whether sought from an adult or adolescent that has the right to give consent, includes specific elements to comply with the obligation that it must:

- Include description of the procedure in simple terms
- Include disclosure of the benefits/adverse risks of the proposed treatment specific to that procedure
- Include evidence-based alternative treatments
- Include disclosure of benefits/adverse risks to the proposed treatment
- Be freely given

A dentist seeking informed consent may view the parent or legal guardian as the only individual who can provide consent for a patient younger than 18 years. This view is a strict interpretation of the laws and constructs of informed consent; however, depending on the state and the situation, in practice the adolescent can be deemed able to render consent.

Many pediatric experts think that, for children as young as age 7 years, effort should be made to include the child in the decision-making process. "A developmental approach to assent anticipates different levels of understanding from children as they age. Providing disclosure of appropriate diagnostic and treatment information and allowing choices about aspects of care, when possible, should be a consistent part of the care plan for children."[5]

Dental providers must show that the care provided and that the options provided for informed consent meet the standard of care, which requires providers to deliver care options consistent with what a reasonably prudent dentist would provide in the same or similar circumstances. Depending on the state, the standard for informed consent could be different. The breadth and depth of the information provided should be consistent with what a reasonably similarly situated patient and reasonably similarly situated prudent practitioner would think necessary to make an appropriate decision. Dentist who do not meet the standard of care may be guilty of negligence. The information should be presented in a manner the patient and responsible adult can understand. Documentation of the informed consent process should be in writing. It is advised that the responsible adult signs the documentation of the informed consent process as evidence to document the process. The risks of nontreatment must be carefully documented and explained in a manner consistent with the cognitive level of the patient and the responsible adult. Requiring the responsible adult to sign a statement acknowledging informed refusal of treatment is recommended.

It should be noted that laws vary related to the age of consent for minors, and the rules governing consent for the treatment of minors are determined by state law. Most states currently have laws that give minors the right to consent to treatment in specific situations. Depending on the state, minors may be allowed to legally consent to treatment of sexually transmitted diseases, birth control, pregnancy, mental health, and substance abuse. In addition, these states often protect as confidential information related to treatment of sexually transmitted diseases, birth control, pregnancy, mental health, and substance abuse. Practitioners should be familiar with the laws governing consent within their jurisdictions. Whenever an adolescent is accompanied by an individual who is not the parent or legal guardian, a provider should be cautious in allowing that individual (eg, a grandparent) to give consent without appropriate documentation.

Based on the circumstances and the urgency of the situation, exceptions to the laws regarding consent allow for emergency care without specific parental consent. Different situations may also allow for the minor to legally consent for their own medical decisions. This provision may include court-ordered emancipation for a child less than 18 years old who lives without parental support and makes day-to-day decisions. In this case, the emancipated minor holds the same legal rights as an adult. Situational emancipation may result from marriage, being a parent, and being a member of the military, and such individuals can consent to their care. Some states use the term emancipated minor.

Because of their ability to drive or use public transportation, adolescents may arrive for a dental appointment without a parent or guardian. A dentist is obligated to get consent from the parent/guardian for dental procedures. This consent can be accomplished via a phone call or Zoom meeting if available. A witness, such as a dental assistant, should be available to hear the discussion and confirmation of consent.

The office should develop clear policy and educate patients about policy and procedures for the care of minors, including the parent/guardian obligation to be present in the office. For example, a policy should clearly state that, for patients between the ages of 12 and 17 years, a parent cannot drop the child off and leave the office, or the parent/legal guardian, if allowed to leave the office, must (1) be available by phone, (2) sign all required documentation, (3) allow only routine treatment.

Informed refusal is a decision by a patient or the parent/legal guardian to decline treatment. The process of informed refusal parallels informed consent, with similar elements required. It is advisable to document refusal of treatment, referral, preventive measures, restorations, and other suggestions made by the provider.

Decision Making and Adolescent Patients

Decision making concerning a patient's care is a responsibility shared by a dentist and the parent or legal guardian. The objective is the best interest of the patient. Dentists should be aware of child-rearing practices that religious, social, and cultural differences may influence. There should also be an awareness that parents may breach their obligations, resulting in child abuse and neglect.

As a minor, an adolescent may not have achieved emancipated status. Decision making about care should include the assent of the patient to the greatest extent possible with the participation of the parents/legal guardian and providers. Consent is given by individuals who have reached the legal age, whereas assent is the agreement of someone not able to give legal consent. Dentists are advised to give serious consideration to each patient's developing capacities during adolescence to participate in decision making, including rationality and autonomy. Providers may not be legally allowed to solicit consent from a minor; however, involving the minor in the discussion about care fosters a stronger provider-patient relationship. Assent can be determined through verbal and nonverbal conduct. When working with adolescents, assent should include at least the following elements:

- Helping the patient achieve a developmentally appropriate awareness of the nature of the condition
- Telling the patient what to expect with the treatment
- Making a clinical assessment of the patient's understanding of the situation and the factors influencing how the patient is responding
- Soliciting an expression of the patient's willingness to accept the proposed care

The Health Insurance Portability and Accountability Act

A parent or legal guardian or other person authorized by a state has the right to an adolescent's medical information. However, if the minor has the right to health care under the state or other law or decision, the minor has an exclusive right to control access to health care information related to the care. A parent can also agree to a confidential agreement between a provider and a minor and then the parent has no right to the information. This situation may frequently occur between a health care provider (eg, physician) and minor. A provider may refuse to provide a parent/legal guardian with information in situations of domestic violence, abuse, or neglect or where the minor could be endangered. However, even in these exceptional situations, the parent may have access to the medical records of the minor related to this treatment when state or other applicable law requires or permits such parental access. If the state or other applicable law is silent on a parent's right of access in these cases, the licensed health care provider may exercise professional judgment to the extent allowed by law to grant or deny parental access to the minor's medical information.

The Privacy Rule generally allows parents to have access to the medical records about their children as their minor children's representatives when such access is not inconsistent with state or other law. There are 3 situations in which the parent would not be the minor's representative under the Privacy Rule. These exceptions are:

- When the minor is the one who consents to care and the consent of the parent is not required under state or other applicable law
- When the minor obtains care at the direction of a court or a person appointed by the court
- When, and to the extent that, the parent agrees that the minor and the health care provider may have a confidential relationship

Dental practitioners should also be aware that the Health Insurance Portability and Accountability Act (HIPAA) Privacy Rule does not cover any health information provided as part of an educational health screening for athletic participation or preenrollment screening. Rules governing access to medical records for adolescents and the protections against disclosure for pregnancy status and sexually transmitted diseases are not afforded the same protection under the Family Educational Rights and Privacy Act (FERPA), a federal law enacted in 1974 that protects the privacy of student education records.

Risky Behaviors

Adolescence is associated with an increased incidence of risk-taking behaviors. Dentists should be aware of the risk-taking behaviors in adolescent patients and monitor current trends or fads. A careful examination of the patient, including a dental and health history, may assist the dentist in identifying such behaviors. The patient may not feel comfortable admitting any of the following behaviors. However, signs and symptoms of such behaviors may be evident to the dentist or a staff member; for example, staining, broken teeth, sudden increase in caries rates, and/or sexually transmitted infections. The dental team should discuss how best to address the issues with the patient and/or the parent and legal guardian. Current trends include:

- Tobacco use
- Alcohol and binge drinking
- Unhealthy dietary practices
- Adolescent sexual activity
- Dating violence
- Substance abuse
- Mental health issues
- Oral piercing
- Weapons possession

Dental patients often develop a relationship of trust with members of the dental team because of an established long-term relationship. During treatment, certain disclosures may reveal risky behaviors on the part of the adolescent patient. The dental team must be prepared to address and respond to any of these situations.

Bullying and Cyberbullying

There has been increased attention to bullying and cyberbullying in the media. The World Health Organization (WHO) and the United Nations recognize bullying as a global health challenge. Bullying is often associated with repeated, intentional, and targeted behavior seeking to intimidate or marginalize someone. Bullying is common and widespread, with the National Center for Educational Statistics reporting that 1 out of 5 students report being bullied.[6] Cyberbullying is using a digital device to send, post, or share negative, mean, or false content, with the same intent to intimidate or marginalize another.

Dental practices often have long-standing relationships with patients and can often detect signs of emotional abuse and neglect. Although the strength of the association is in debate, children with observable dental problems and malocclusions have an increased incidence of bullying and emotional abuse.[7] Whether it is from within the child's home environment or from the child's social circle or at school, dental practitioners have an ethical obligation to be alert to the signs and symptoms of emotional abuse associated with bullying.

The common signs of emotional abuse include a lack of interest in conversation, weight loss, unwillingness to participate in activities, and poor academic performance. It is important ethically to educate members of the dental team to recognize the signs and symptoms of bullying.

Pregnant Adolescent Patients

Patients may disclose to a dental provider their pregnancies. Dentists may be presented with an ethical dilemma when a patient requests that the parent or guardian not be informed. The dentist needs to weigh the issues and decide about the next steps. From an ethical and legal viewpoint, the patient and their fetus need to be protected and cared for, thus informing a parent or guardian may be the appropriate step. However, providers should talk with the patient to make sure that the patient is not put in harm's way because of the disclosure, and, instead of informing the parent, protective child services may need to be contacted. The situations that could trigger contacting an external agency include the pregnancy resulting from a parent or someone in the household sexually abusing the patient, or patients feeling that they will be in danger if the pregnancy is reported. It is the obligation of the provider to get information about the patient and the personal circumstances before deciding whether to inform the parent/legal guardian or choose another option.

Tooth Whitening

Adolescent patients and their parents may request specific procedures that the dental provider may or may not be comfortable doing. Adolescent patients often have an increased self-awareness of their appearance and often express interest in cosmetic procedures. Professional associations offer guidance to providers. The American Academy of Pediatric Dentistry discourages full-arch cosmetic bleaching for child and adolescent patients in the mixed dentition and primary dentition. (https://www.aapd.org/globalassets/media/publications/archives/lee-27-5.pdf).

Current Trends and Issues

To satisfy dental providers' legal and ethical obligations, dentists need to be cognizant of current trends and issues as health care providers.

Child abuse and neglect

There is an ethical and legal obligation to report suspected abuse and neglect. Dental providers should use their training in identifying mistreatment and be familiar with the agencies responsible for child protection and the process for reporting.

Human trafficking

Human trafficking is a criminal human rights violation and significant health issue. Many jurisdictions require that dental professionals report suspected human trafficking. Trafficking frequently occurs in women, children, and adolescents. Education about the signs of trafficking and protocol for reporting are important to know.

Responsible opioid prescribing

Dental practitioners have a legal and ethical duty to manage patient discomfort responsibly. Increasing evidence suggests that dental prescribing of opioids contributes to addiction and abuse behaviors. In addition, the Drug Enforcement Agency has enhanced its enforcement efforts against dentists who are prescribing without documented medical necessity. Many states have laws and regulations regarding the prescribing of controlled substances and specific registration requirements.

Gender Identity/Transitioning Patients

A 2017 University of California, Los Angeles, study estimated that 0.7% of teenagers aged 13–17 years identify as transgender.[8] That translates to 150,000 teenagers nationally. A subsequent Minnesota study of ninth and eleventh graders found that 2.7% identified as transgender or gender nonconforming.[9] The Centers for Disease Control and Prevention (CDC) reports that nearly 2% of high school students identify as transgender.[10]

Regardless of the exact number, dentists need to be aware and responsive to the needs and issues associated with gender identity and gender nonconformity. Patients who are expressing transgender identities and gender nonconformity are more likely to have depression and engage in other risky behaviors.

Transgender teenagers also show oral sequelae, including oral manifestations from pharmaceutical drugs and poor dietary and eating habits. Dental teams have an ethical responsibility to adequately educate themselves on the needs of transgender adolescents and prepare themselves to accommodate and support the patients' emotional and psychological expression of their identities.

SUMMARY

There are many complicated legal and ethical issues that dental practitioners encounter when caring for adolescent patients. The dental team should understand the scope of responsibilities and develop clear and consistent policies and practices to respond to the issues encountered.

CLINICS CARE POINTS

- Patient involvement in the informed consent process for dental care in adolescent patients should be relative to their physical, psychosocial, and cognitive development, and certain aspects of the medical history may be deemed confidential and not accessible by the parent/guardian.

- Medically and legally, the provider should be familiar with the specific requirements for documentation relative to each individual insurance plan and Medicaid agreement, and, in particular, the chart notes should carefully document the existing conditions, medical necessity for treatment, and the specifics of treatment provided.

- Because adolescents are a vulnerable population, dental providers should understand their legal responsibilities for identifying and reporting evidence of child abuse, neglect, and human trafficking, and have an ethical responsibility to identify mental health issues and issues associated with patients who are being bullied.

- The American Academy of Pediatric Dentistry is the recognized association for the specialty of pediatric dentistry, and offers extensive materials for the management and treatment of adolescent patients. Practitioners should familiarize themselves with the guidelines for adolescent dental care as a reference point for the standard of care for the management of adolescent patients.

- Careful attention to the informed consent process improves communication between the patients and their parents/guardians. Clear documentation, a process for dealing with unaccompanied teenagers, and a systematic method of addressing changes in the treatment plan and posttreatment communication are important.

DISCLOSURE

The authors have nothing to disclose.

REFERENCES

1. American Academy of Pediatric Dentistry Policy on Patient's Bill of Rights and Responsibilities. Available at: https://www.aapd.org/research/oral-health-policies–recommendations/patients-bill-of-rights-and-responsibilities/. Accessed April 16, 2021.
2. American Academy of Pediatrics. Adolescent Sexual Health. Stages of Adolescent Development. Available at: https://www.aap.org/en-us/advocacy-and-policy/aap-health-initiatives/adolescent-sexual-health/Pages/Stages-of-Adolescent-Development.aspx. Accessed April 21, 2021.
3. American Dental Association. Principles of Ethics and Code of Professional Conduct. With official advisory opinions revised to November 2020. Available at: https://www.ada.org/~/media/ADA/Member%20Center/Ethics/ADA_Code_Of_Ethics_November_2020.pdf?la=en. Accessed April 16, 2021.
4. 20 Medicaid & CHIP Enrollment Data Highlights. Available at: https://www.medicaid.gov/medicaid/program-information/medicaid-and-chip-enrollment-data/report-highlights/index.html. Accessed April 20, 2021.
5. Informed Consent in Decision-Making in Pediatric Practice. Committee on Bioethics, American Academy of Pediatrics. Available at: https://pediatrics.aappublications.org/content/pediatrics/138/2/e20161484.full.pdf. Accessed April 19, 2021.
6. Student Reports of Bullying: Results from the 2017 School Crime Supplement to the National Crime Victimization Survey. U.S. Department of Education. Available at: https://nces.ed.gov/pubs2019/2019054.pdf. Accessed April 30, 2021.
7. Seehra J, Fleming PS, Newton T, et al. Bullying in orthodontic patients and its relationship to malocclusion, self-esteem and oral health-related quality of life. J Orthod 2011;38:247–56 [quiz: 294].
8. Age of Individuals Who Identify as Transgender in the United States. Available at: https://williamsinstitute.law.ucla.edu/publications/age-trans-individuals-us/%20UCLA%20School%20of%20Law%20Williams%20Institute. Accessed April 29, 2021.
9. Eisenberg ME, Gower AL, McMorris BJ, et al. Risk and Protective Factors in the Lives of Transgender/Gender Nonconforming Adolescents. J Adolesc Health 2017;61:521–6.
10. Youth Risk Behavior Survey Data Summary and Trends Report 2007–2017. Available at: https://www.cdc.gov/healthyyouth/data/yrbs/pdf/trendsreport.pdf. Accessed April 29, 2021.

UNITED STATES POSTAL SERVICE ®

Statement of Ownership, Management, and Circulation
(All Periodicals Publications Except Requester Publications)

1. Publication Title	2. Publication Number	3. Filing Date
DENTAL CLINICS OF NORTH AMERICA	566 – 480	9/18/2021

4. Issue Frequency	5. Number of Issues Published Annually	6. Annual Subscription Price
JAN, APR, JUL, OCT	4	$313.00

7. Complete Mailing Address of Known Office of Publication (Not printer) (Street, city, county, state, and ZIP+4®)

ELSEVIER INC.
230 Park Avenue, Suite 800
New York, NY 10169

Contact Person
Malathi Samayan

Telephone (Include area code)
91-44-4299-4507

8. Complete Mailing Address of Headquarters or General Business Office of Publisher (Not printer)

ELSEVIER INC.
230 Park Avenue, Suite 800
New York, NY 10169

9. Full Names and Complete Mailing Addresses of Publisher, Editor, and Managing Editor (Do not leave blank)

Publisher (Name and complete mailing address)

Dolores Meloni, ELSEVIER INC.
1600 JOHN F KENNEDY BLVD, SUITE 1800
PHILADELPHIA, PA 19103-2899

Editor (Name and complete mailing address)

JOHN VASSALLO, ELSEVIER INC.
1600 JOHN F KENNEDY BLVD, SUITE 1800
PHILADELPHIA, PA 19103-2899

Managing Editor (Name and complete mailing address)

PATRICK MANLEY, ELSEVIER INC.
1600 JOHN F KENNEDY BLVD, SUITE 1800
PHILADELPHIA, PA 19103-2899

10. Owner (Do not leave blank. If the publication is owned by a corporation, give the name and address of the corporation immediately followed by the names and addresses of all stockholders owning or holding 1 percent or more of the total amount of stock. If not owned by a corporation, give the names and addresses of the individual owners. If owned by a partnership or other unincorporated firm, give its name and address as well as those of each individual owner. If the publication is published by a nonprofit organization, give its name and address.)

Full Name	Complete Mailing Address
WHOLLY OWNED SUBSIDIARY OF REED/ELSEVIER, US HOLDINGS	1600 JOHN F KENNEDY BLVD, SUITE 1800 PHILADELPHIA, PA 19103-2899

11. Known Bondholders, Mortgagees, and Other Security Holders Owning or Holding 1 Percent or More of Total Amount of Bonds, Mortgages, or Other Securities. If none, check box → ☐ None

Full Name	Complete Mailing Address
N/A	

12. Tax Status (For completion by nonprofit organizations authorized to mail at nonprofit rates) (Check one)
The purpose, function, and nonprofit status of this organization and the exempt status for federal income tax purposes:
☒ Has Not Changed During Preceding 12 Months
☐ Has Changed During Preceding 12 Months (Publisher must submit explanation of change with this statement)

PS Form 3526, July 2014 [Page 1 of 4 (see instructions page 4)] PSN: 7530-01-000-9931   PRIVACY NOTICE: See our privacy policy on www.usps.com.

---

13. Publication Title			14. Issue Date for Circulation Data Below
DENTAL CLINICS OF NORTH AMERICA			JULY 2021

15. Extent and Nature of Circulation			Average No. Copies Each Issue During Preceding 12 Months	No. Copies of Single Issue Published Nearest to Filing Date
a. Total Number of Copies (Net press run)			250	226
b. Paid Circulation (By Mail and Outside the Mail)	(1)	Mailed Outside-County Paid Subscriptions Stated on PS Form 3541 (Include paid distribution above nominal rate, advertiser's proof copies, and exchange copies)	140	125
	(2)	Mailed In-County Paid Subscriptions Stated on PS Form 3541 (Include paid distribution above nominal rate, advertiser's proof copies, and exchange copies)	0	0
	(3)	Paid Distribution Outside the Mails Including Sales Through Dealers and Carriers, Street Vendors, Counter Sales, and Other Paid Distribution Outside USPS®	87	62
	(4)	Paid Distribution by Other Classes of Mail Through the USPS (e.g., First-Class Mail®)	0	0
c. Total Paid Distribution [Sum of 15b (1), (2), (3), and (4)]			227	187
d. Free or Nominal Rate Distribution (By Mail and Outside the Mail)	(1)	Free or Nominal Rate Outside-County Copies included on PS Form 3541	20	22
	(2)	Free or Nominal Rate In-County Copies Included on PS Form 3541	0	0
	(3)	Free or Nominal Rate Copies Mailed at Other Classes Through the USPS (e.g., First-Class Mail)	0	0
	(4)	Free or Nominal Rate Distribution Outside the Mail (Carriers or other means)	0	0
e. Total Free or Nominal Rate Distribution (Sum of 15d (1), (2), (3) and (4))			20	22
f. Total Distribution (Sum of 15c and 15e)			247	209
g. Copies not Distributed (See Instructions to Publishers #4 (page #3))			15	17
h. Total (Sum of 15f and g)			261	226
i. Percent Paid (15c divided by 15f times 100)			91.90%	89.47%

* If you are claiming electronic copies, go to line 16 on page 3. If you are not claiming electronic copies, skip to line 17 on page 3.

PS Form 3526, July 2014 (Page 2 of 4)

16. Electronic Copy Circulation	Average No. Copies Each Issue During Preceding 12 Months	No. Copies of Single Issue Published Nearest to Filing Date
a. Paid Electronic Copies	▲	
b. Total Paid Print Copies (Line 15c) + Paid Electronic Copies (Line 16a)	▲	
c. Total Print Distribution (Line 15f) + Paid Electronic Copies (Line 16a)	▲	
d. Percent Paid (Both Print & Electronic Copies) (16b divided by 16c × 100)		

☒ I certify that 50% of all my distributed copies (electronic and print) are paid above a nominal price.

17. Publication of Statement of Ownership

☒ If the publication is a general publication, publication of this statement is required. Will be printed in the ____OCTOBER 2021____ issue of this publication.   ☐ Publication not required.

18. Signature and Title of Editor, Publisher, Business Manager, or Owner

Malathi Samayan

Malathi Samayan - Distribution Controller

Date
9/18/2021

I certify that all information furnished on this form is true and complete. I understand that anyone who furnishes false or misleading information on this form or who omits material or information requested on the form may be subject to criminal sanctions (including fines and imprisonment) and/or civil sanctions (including civil penalties).

PS Form 3526, July 2014 (Page 3 of 4)   PRIVACY NOTICE: See our privacy policy on www.usps.com

Moving?

Make sure your subscription moves with you!

To notify us of your new address, find your **Clinics Account Number** (located on your mailing label above your name), and contact customer service at:

Email: journalscustomerservice-usa@elsevier.com

800-654-2452 (subscribers in the U.S. & Canada)
314-447-8871 (subscribers outside of the U.S. & Canada)

Fax number: 314-447-8029

Elsevier Health Sciences Division
Subscription Customer Service
3251 Riverport Lane
Maryland Heights, MO 63043

*To ensure uninterrupted delivery of your subscription, please notify us at least 4 weeks in advance of move.